PRE-CLINICAL MEDICINE
SAQs, MCQs and EMQs

PRE-CLINICAL MEDICINE
SAQs, MCQs and EMQs

Calver Pang

Johns Hopkins University School of Medicine

Ibraz Hussain

University Hospitals of Leicester

John Mayberry

University Hospitals of Leicester

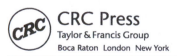

CRC Press
Taylor & Francis Group
Boca Raton London New York

CRC Press is an imprint of the
Taylor & Francis Group, an **informa** business

CRC Press
Taylor & Francis Group
6000 Broken Sound Parkway NW, Suite 300
Boca Raton, FL 33487-2742

© 2018 by Taylor & Francis Group, LLC
CRC Press is an imprint of Taylor & Francis Group, an Informa business

No claim to original U.S. Government works

Printed on acid-free paper

International Standard Book Number-13: 978-1-138-06611-3 (Hardback)
978-1-138-06609-0 (Paperback)

Library of Congress Cataloging-in-Publication Data

Names: Pang, Calver, author. | Hussain, Ibraz, author. | Mayberry, John F., author.
Title: Pre-clinical medicine : SAQs, MCQs and EMQs / Calver Pang, Ibraz Hussain,
John Francis Mayberry.
Description: Boca Raton : CRC Press, [2018]
Identifiers: LCCN 2017023818 (print) | LCCN 2017024706 (ebook) |
ISBN 9781315159317 (Master eBook) | ISBN 9781138066090 (pbk. : alk. paper) |
ISBN 9781138066113 (hardback : alk. paper)
Subjects: | MESH: Signs and Symptoms | Diagnosis, Differential | Anatomy |
Physiological Phenomena | Examination Questions | Case Reports
Classification: LCC RC71.3 (ebook) | LCC RC71.3 (print) | NLM WB 18.2 | DDC
616.07/5076--dc23
LC record available at https://lccn.loc.gov/2017023818

Visit the Taylor & Francis Web site at
http://www.taylorandfrancis.com

and the CRC Press Web site at
http://www.crcpress.com

Contents

Preface

Over the past few years, medical school exams have changed dramatically in an attempt to imitate the style of postgraduate exams. Many question and answer books that have been released have primarily focused on clinical medicine and are aimed at final-year students.

The road toward qualification as a junior doctor is paved with a long series of assessments and exams. As junior doctors, we are aware of the tendency medical students have to concentrate on clinical medicine, as it is most relevant and most interesting. However, it is essential that a good foundation on basic sciences is developed before proceeding onto the clinical components of medicine. That is why we felt it was vital for students to have access to high-quality practice questions to aid learning in pre-clinical medicine and provide feedback.

In this book, we have produced questions and answers on pre-clinical medicine covering the core areas of each organ system. The aim is to integrate other disciplines of medicine with each question to encourage application of knowledge. We have endeavoured to make this book a useful resource for exam revision in the pre-clinical phase. We hope this book will provide you with the information required en route to the successful completion of the pre-clinical phase of medical school.

Calver Pang and Ibraz Hussain

Acknowledgements

First and foremost, we thank Professor John Mayberry for encouraging and guiding us in writing this book. We especially thank Angie Gillies and the Core Biotechnology Services from the University of Leicester in obtaining the histology slides. We wish to thank Dr. John Le Quesne and Dr. Madhumita Das for producing the images of the histology slides required for publication and Dr. Ana Gonzalez and Professor Giles Perryer for their kind permission to use the images on page 9 and page 48. We thank Lei Ka Pou for her illustrations in this book.

We thank our families and friends for their support and patience while we were writing this book. Finally, Dr. Calver Pang would like to thank his mentor Dr. John Harmon.

Authors

Calver Pang MBChB MPharm (Hons) is a Foundation Year 2 Doctor in the Yorkshire and Humber Deanery. He holds a surgical research fellowship from Johns Hopkins University School of Medicine and is an active researcher specialising in wound healing.

In his medical career, he has published in numerous peer-reviewed journals and presented nationally and internationally on a wide range of topics. He has a long-term aspiration of becoming an academic plastic surgeon.

Ibraz Hussain MBChB BSc (Hons) practiced as an audiologist in the NHS before going on to study medicine. He is currently a Foundation Year 2 Doctor in the East Midlands Deanery.

He has a strong interest in medical education and mentoring, and hopes to combine this with his future plans to train in general practice.

John Mayberry DSc MD LLM MSc (medical education) is a consultant physician and professor of gastroenterology in Leicester. His main interests are in the epidemiology of chronic gastrointestinal diseases and in the equitable delivery of health care.

Abbreviations

AAA	abdominal aortic aneurysm	CFTR	Cystic fibrosis transmembrane conductance regulator
Ab	antibody		
ABPI	ankle brachial pressure index	cGMP	cyclic guanosine monophosphate
ACE	angiotensin converting enzyme	CHD	congenital hip dysplasia
		CNS	central nervous system
ACEi	angiotensin converting enzyme inhibitor	COCP	combined oral contraceptive pill
ACh	acetylcholine	COPD	chronic obstructive pulmonary disease
AChE	acetylcholinesterase		
AChR	acetylcholine receptor	CSF	cerebrospinal fluid
ACS	acute coronary syndrome	CT	computed tomography
ACTH	adrenocorticotrophic hormone	CTPA	computed tomography pulmonary angiogram
ADH	antidiuretic hormone	CXR	chest xray
ADP	adenosine diphosphate	DMD	Duchenne muscular dystrophy
A&E	accident and emergency		
AF	atrial fibrillation	DNA	Deoxyribonucleic acid
AKI	acute kidney injury	DVT	deep vein thrombosis
ANS	autonomic nervous system	EBV	Epstein barr virus
ALP	alkaline phosphatase	ECG	electrocardiogram
ALT	alanine transaminase	eGFR	estimated glomerular filtration rate
APTT	activated partial thromboplastin time	FEV1	forced expiratory volume in 1 second
AR	aortic regurgitation		
AS	aortic stenosis	FVC	forced vital capacity
AST	aspartate transaminase	FSH	follicle stimulating hormone
ATP	adenosine triphosphate		
AXR	abdominal x-ray	FDP	flexor digitorum profundus
BBB	bundle branch block		
BMI	body mass index	FPL	flexor pollicis longus
BP	blood pressure	GCS	Glasgow coma score
bpm	beats per minute	GP	general practice, general practitioner
CABG	coronary artery bypass graft		
		HAP	hospital acquired pneumonia
CAD	coronary artery disease		
cAMP	cyclic adenosine monophosphate	Hb	haemoglobin
		hCG	human chorionic gonadotrophine
CAP	community acquired pneumonia	HIV	human immunodeficiency virus
CBD	common bile duct		
CF	cystic fibrosis	HPV	human papilloma virus

HSV	herpes simplex virus	OSA	obstructive sleep apnoea
HUS	Haemolytic uraemic syndrome	pANCA	perinuclear anti-neutrophil cytoplasmic antibodies
IL	interleukin		
ITU	intensive treatment unit	PCI	primary coronary intervention
IVC	inferior vena cava		
JVP	jugular venous pressure	PCOS	polycystic ovary syndrome
K+	potassium	PCR	Polymerase chain reaction
LDH	Lactate dehydrogenase	PDA	patent ductus arteriosus
LH	luteinising hormone	PE	pulmonary embolism
LMN	lower motor neurone	PID	pelvic inflammatory disease
LMWH	low molecular weight heparin	PKP	Phosphofructokinase
LUQ	left upper quadrant	PPI	proton pump inhibitor
LV	left ventricle, left ventricular	PR	per rectum
		PSA	prostate specific antigen
LVH	left ventricular hypertrophy	PTH	parathyroid hormone
		PVD	peripheral vascular disease
MCA	middle cerebral artery	RA	rheumatoid arthritis
MCP	metacarpophalangeal	RBC	red blood cell
M,C&S	microscopy, culture & sensitivity	RNA	ribonucleic acid
		RR	respiratory rate
MCV	mean cell volume	RUQ	right upper quadrant
MCH	mean cell haemoglobin	RV	right ventricle, right ventricular
MI	myocardial infarction		
MND	motor neurone disease	RVH	right ventricular hypertrophy
MR	mitral regurgitation		
MRI	magnetic resonance imaging	SA	sinoatrial
		SAH	subarachnoid haemorrhage
MS	multiple sclerosis		
MSU	midstream urine	SDS-PAGE	Sodium dodecyl sulfate polyacrylamide gel electrophoresis
mV	millivolt		
Na	sodium		
NaCl	sodium chloride	SIADH	syndrome of inappropriate antidiuretic hormone secretion
NG	nasogastric		
NICE	National institute of health and clinical excellence		
		SLE	systemic lupus erythematous
NIV	non-invasive ventilation	SOB	shortness of breath
NPH	normal pressure hydrocephalus	SSRI	selective serotonin reuptake inhibitor
NSAID	non-steroidal anti-inflammatory drug	STEMI	ST segment elevation myocardial infarction
OA	osteoarthritis	SVC	superior vena cava
OGD	oesophago-gastroduodenoscopy	SVT	supraventricular tachycardia

TB	tuberculosis	UC	ulcerative colitis
TIA	transient ischaemic attack	U&Es	urea and electrolytes
TOF	Tetralogy of Fallot	UFH	unfractionated heparin
TSH	thyroid stimulating hormone	UMN	upper motor neurone
		USS	ultrasound scan
TURP	transurethral resection of the prostate	UTI	urinary tract infection
		VZV	varicella zoster virus
T3	Triiodothyronine	WCC	white cell count
T4	Thyroxine		

Blood test reference ranges

Haematology

Haemoglobin	130–180 g/L (adult male)
	115–170 g/L (adult female)
Mean cell volume (MCV)	80–100 f/L
Mean cell haemoglobin (MCH)	27–32 pg
Platelet count	150–400 × 10⁹/L
White cell count	3.5–11 × 10⁹/L
Neutrophils	1.8–7.5 × 10⁹/L
Eosinophils	0.1–0.4 × 10⁹/L
Basophils	0.02–0.1 × 10⁹/L
C-reactive protein (CRP)	<10 mg/L

Coagulation

International normalized ratio (INR)	0.9–1.2
Activated partial thromboplastin time (aPTT)	20–40 secs

Haematinics

Ferritin	10–300 ng/mL
Vitamin B12	180–1000 pg/mL
Folate	>4 ng/mL

Electrolytes

Sodium	133–146 mmol/L
Potassium	3.5–5.3 mmol/L
Urea	2.5–7.8 mmol/L
Creatinine	0.8–1.3 mg/d
eGFR	>90

Bone profile

Serum Phosphate	0.8–1.5 mmol/L
Serum Magnesium	0.7–1.0 mmol/L
Total calcium	2–2.6 mmol/L

Lipids

Triglycerides	50–150 mg/dL
Total cholesterol	3–5.5 mmol/L

Liver function tests

Albumin	35–50 g/L
Bilirubin	3–17 μmol/L
Alkaline phosphatase	50–100 U/L
Alanine aminotransferase (ALT)	5–30 U/L
Amylase	30–125 U/L
Aspartate aminotransferase (AST)	5–30 U/L
Gamma glutamyl transferase (GGT)	6–50 U/L

Miscellaneous

HbA1c	4%–6% (20–42 IFCC)
TSH	0.4–4.0 mIU/L
Free T4	9.0–25 pmol/L
Creatine kinase	40–320 U/L (male)
	25–200 U/L (female)

Acid Base

pH	7.35–7.45
Base excess	(–2)–(+2)
H+	36–44 nmol/L
Partial pressure of oxygen (PaO$_2$)	>10.6 kPa (75–100 mmHg)
Oxygen saturation	96%–100%
Partial pressure of carbon dioxide (PaCO$_2$)	4.7–6 kPa (35–45 mm Hg)
Bicarbonate (HCO$_3$)	18–22 mmol/L

Chapter 1

CELLULAR STRUCTURE AND FUNCTION

1. A young girl is on the ward with a history of long bone fractures resulting from only minor injuries. Her sclerae appears blue, her skin is hyperextensible and she has difficulty in hearing.
   a. Name two important functions of collagen (1)
   b. Why can disorders of collagen affect so many tissues? (1)
   c. Explain the effects of dietary deficiency of vitamin C on collagen (2)
   d. Inherited collagen disorders commonly show a dominant pattern of inheritance. Explain this observation (1)
   e. Collagen has an abnormally high content of glycine and proline. Explain the importance of these amino acids to the structure of collagen (2)
   f. Name three post-translational modifications that collagen undergoes during its synthesis, indicating whether they occur intracellularly or extracellulary (3)

2. Amylase is a major group of enzymes found in the pancreas and salivary glands. It hydrolyses dietary starch into disaccharides and trisaccharides which are then converted to glucose via different enzymes to provide energy to the body.
   a. Define the term Km (1)
   b. Describe the function of an enzyme 'active site' and briefly explain how features of its structure are related to its function (2)
   c. Define the term allosteric regulation as applied to enzymes (1)
   d. Give an example of an enzyme known to be regulated in an allosteric manner. Indicate two of the regulatory processes concerned, stating whether they are activating or inhibiting (3)
   e. Describe how the effect of one of the allosteric regulatory mechanisms you have mentioned is achieved (3)

3. A 2-year-old boy has been admitted to hospital following recurrent chest infections. One of his parents is known to have cystic fibrosis (CF). A sweat test has been carried out showing a chloride level of 80 mmol/L. A diagnosis of CF has been made.
   a. What type of inherited condition is CF? (1)
   b. If two parents both with CF are to have children, what is the probability that the child will also have CF? (1)
   c. What exactly is the protein deficiency in people with CF? Explain the consequences of this (3)
   d. How would you screen for CF carriers? (1)
   e. Name four symptoms of CF (2)
   f. Why are people with CF more likely to develop respiratory infection? (1)
   g. What is meant by gene penetrance? (1)

4. James, a 5-year-old boy, has been complaining of leg cramps. His mother takes him to see his GP. He is suspected to have Duchenne muscular dystrophy (DMD).
   a. What is the pattern of inheritance for DMD? (1)
   b. The mutation rate in the DMD gene is relatively high. What is the most likely explanation for this? (1)
   c. Given that James' mother is not a carrier, provide two possible genetic explanations for James inheriting the mutation. For each explanation, include an estimation of the risk of recurrence of DMD in future offspring (2)
   d. What are the three main types of muscle tissue? Give a histologically distinguishing feature for each type (3)
   e. Name three specific biochemical markers which indicate muscle damage (1)
   f. What reaction does creatine kinase catalyse and what is the importance of this? (2)

5. Ms. J. G., an 18-year-old African-Caribbean girl, goes to her GP complaining of tiredness and lethargy. Investigations show that she has iron deficiency anaemia.
   a. Name two possible causes of iron deficiency anaemia (1)
   b. Concerning erythropoiesis, where does it occur? Give two cofactors that are required (2)
   c. On the graph below, draw and label an oxygen dissociation curve for foetal haemoglobin and myoglobin (2)

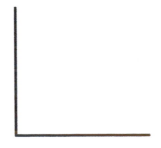

   d. Explain how the oxygen dissociation curve for Hb is related to its molecular structure, and how the oxygen dissociation curve for myoglobin relates to its structure (2)
   e. Give three factors that affect the oxygen dissociation curve for haemoglobin and give the effect(s) of each (3)

6. A young girl with known Ehlers–Danlos syndrome presents to A&E with a left elbow dislocation. Below is a diagram of a sodium dodecyl sulfate polyacrylamide gel electrophoresis (SDS–PAGE) showing type III collagen in this patient.

a. Which protein has higher molecular weight and why? (2)

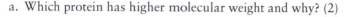
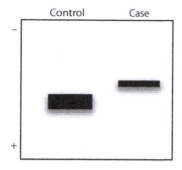

The site at which the restriction enzyme acts was mutated in the patient. This enzyme has a 110 base sequence. This sequence was amplified by polymerase chain reaction (PCR) from a normal individual and the patient, digested by the restriction enzyme. The normal individual shows two bands of size 70 base pairs and 40 base pairs.

b. Indicate the expected band size if the mutated strip was put into a solution with restriction enzymes, and why (2)
c. What is the key property of tropocollagen and how does this benefit the function of collagen? (2)
d. What is the function of hydroxyapatite in bone? (1)
e. Which cells form collagen in bone? (1)
f. Which cells form collagen in cartilage? (1)
g. Which type of cartilage forms the epiglottis? (1)

7. Male aged 18 years has a partner who is 15 weeks pregnant, with a baby of unknown gender. He is known to have sickle cell trait. His father had sickle cell anaemia and his mother was unaffected. His partner is also unaffected. He has a sister who is unaware of whether she has sickle cell trait or not. Her husband and her two daughters are unaffected.
a. What is the inheritance pattern of sickle cell anaemia? (1)
b. What is the base pair mutation in sickle cell anaemia and what is the resultant amino acid change in the β-haemoglobin protein? (2)
c. What are the genotypes for mum and dad of the unborn child using the allele notations Bs for the sickle cell allele, and B for the normal allele? (1)
d. Draw and annotate a pedigree with the information given above (3)
e. Calculate the probability of a child being born with sickle cell naemia if one parent has sickle cell anaemia and the other has sickle cell trait. (1)
f. Give one possible ethical implication to consider prior to genetic testing and potential diagnosis of sickle cell anaemia in the unborn baby for:
   i. the child itself (1)
   ii. the child's parents (1)

MCQ

For the following questions, select the single best answer.

1. A 38-year-old man presents with renal failure. Both his father and his son have the same condition. What is the most likely mode of inheritance?
   a. Autosomal dominant
   b. Autosomal recessive
   c. Mitochondrial
   d. X-linked dominant
   e. X-linked recessive

2. If the total amount of adenine in a double-stranded DNA is 23%, what is the amount of thymine, cytosine, and guanine in this DNA?
   a. 46%, 15.5%, 15.5%
   b. 46%, 23.25%, 7.75%
   c. 23%, 27%, 27%
   d. 23%, 40.5%, 13.5%
   e. None of the above

3. Which of the following statements are true?
   a. The TATA box is located in the exon
   b. The TATA box has the core DNA sequence 5′ TATA 3′
   c. The TATA box is usually located 50 base pairs upstream of transcription site
   d. The TATA box is not transcribed
   e. Ribonucleic acid (RNA) polymerase II binds to TATA box to initiate transcription

4. Which of the following will NOT cause a right shift of the oxygen dissociation curve?
   a. Chronic anaemia
   b. Decrease in blood pH
   c. Increase in tissue temperature
   d. Exercise
   e. All of the above

5. Reverse transcriptase PCR uses which of the following:
   a. DNA as a template to form RNA
   b. Messenger RNA (mRNA) as a template to form complementary DNA (cDNA)
   c. DNA as a template to form single-stranded DNA (ssDNA)
   d. RNA as a template to form micro RNA (miRNA)
   e. None of the above

6. Which of the following condition is NOT an example of compound heterozygosity?
   a. Beta thalassaemia
   b. Phenylketonuria

c. Tay–Sachs disease
d. Cystic fibrosis
e. Huntington's disease

7. What does the following diagram represent?

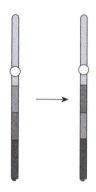

a. Paracentric inversion
b. Reciprocal translocation
c. Pericentric inversion
d. Robertsonian translocation
e. Deletion

EMQ

For each of the following questions, select the most appropriate answer.

Each option may be used once, more than once or not at all.

A. Haemophilia A
B. Vitamin K
C. Tissue factor
D. Factor X
E. Haemophilia B
F. Low-molecular-weight heparin (LMWH)
G. Von Willebrand disease
H. Warfarin
I. Factor V
J. Disseminated intravascular coagulation

8. A 15-year-old girl is brought into your clinic due to increased bleeding following a tooth extraction two days ago. She also complains of heavy periods that typically last for more than five days. On examination you noticed bruising over both arms. Investigation results show increase in activated partial thromboplastin time (APTT) but prothrombin time (PT) and platelets are normal. What is the diagnosis?

9. Which factor initiates the extrinsic pathway?

10. A 60-year-old man complains of sudden dyspnoea and pleuritic chest pain. On examination, BP is 95/60 mmHg and respiratory rate is 32. A D-dimer test is requested and shows it is elevated. What immediate management would you start on this patient?

Chapter 2

BODY TISSUES

1. A 66-year-old man presents to his GP with a dark pigmented lesion on his face. He complains that it is itchy and occasionally bleeds, and states that he rarely uses sun protection.
   a. Below is a histology slide of the skin. Label the dermis, epidermis and sebaceous gland (3)

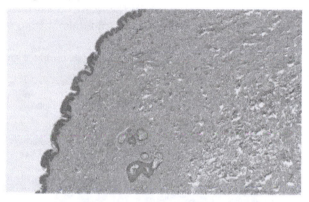

   b. Describe the cycle of epidermal cell differentiation (3)
   c. Name the two most common skin cancers (1)
   d. What is the most important risk factor of skin cancer? (1)
   e. How does this biochemical factor cause skin cancer? (1)
   f. Name two routes in which cancer can spread (1)

2. A 25-year-old is admitted to A&E following a road traffic accident. She has multiple injuries including a laceration to her wrist which has resulted in loss of motor and sensory function.
   a. Label on this diagram the Schwann cell, node of Ranvier, myelin sheath and axon (2)

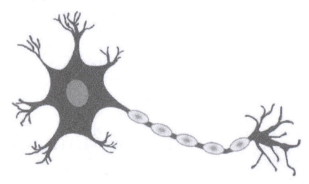

b. Briefly explain the role of Schwann cells in neurotransmission (2)

c. Name and state a function of two neuroglial cell types in the central nervous system (2)

d. Describe the process of Wallerian degeneration (2)

e. According to Seddon's classification, name the three basic types of peripheral nerve injury (1)

f. If a nerve injury at the wrist involved a distance of 90 mm, estimate the number of days required for nerve regeneration (1)

3. At 28 weeks gestation, a woman underwent a routine sonography which showed a large fluid-filled structure within the uterus. A subsequent MRI showed a large cystic mass arising from the sacrococcygeal region of the foetus. The mass had no solid components and there was no involvement of the neural tube.

a. Label the syncytiotrophoblast, cytotrophoblast, epiblast and maternal sinusoid (2)

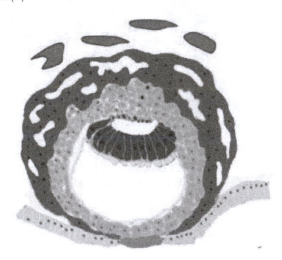

b. Where does implantation occur and by which day is this process completed? (2)

c. Describe the most likely cause for this congenital defect (1)

d. A sample of the mass was taken; which derivatives of the germ layer(s) would you expect to see? (1)

e. Briefly outline how the neural tube is formed (3)

f. Name one example of an open neural tube defect (1)

4. A 52-year-old man presents with sudden onset upper abdominal pain which radiates to the back. Observations show a heart rate of 110 bpm, a respiratory rate of 20 and a temperature 37.5°C. On further questioning you find out that he has a history of high alcohol consumption.

a. Label the islets of Langerhans (1)

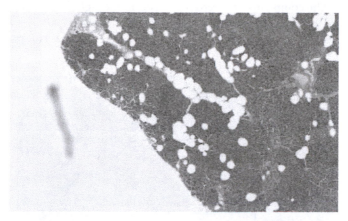

b. Give two examples of secretions from this cell type (2)
c. Describe the process of merocrine secretion and give an example of a gland that uses this mechanism (3)
d. Fill in the following table stating whether the gland is exocrine, endocrine or both (2)

Gonad	
Adrenal	
Parathyroid	
Goblet cell	

On examination he is found to have blue/grey staining around the umbilicus and flanks. A diagnosis of acute pancreatitis is made.

e. What is the significance of the sphincter of Oddi in pancreatitis? (2)

5. A child is referred to a paediatric clinic due to an abnormal gait and poor balance. This child has a family history of muscular dystrophy.
   a. Label the A, I, M, H, and Z bands, and mark the length of a sarcomere (3)

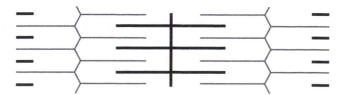

b. What proteins are in the A and I bands? (1)
c. Describe the sequence of events involved in skeletal muscle contraction (4)
d. Troponins are used as a marker in cardiac ischaemia. What is the role of fibroblasts in such event? (2)

6. A 78-year-old woman attends the A&E department following a fall in her garden. She complains of severe pain around the right hip and an X-ray confirms a hip fracture.
   a. Below is a histology slide of a compact bone. Label the Haversian canal and lacunae (2)

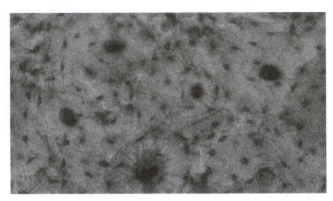

Reproduced with permission of Dr Ana Gonzalez and Prof. Giles Perryer

   b. Why are postmenopausal women are at increased risk of osteoporosis? (2)
   c. Name two other risk factors of osteoporosis (1)
   d. Name a class of drug that is used as a treatment of osteoporosis (1)
   e. Explain the process of fracture healing (4)

MCQ

For the following questions, select the single best answer.

1. What is the process where bone is formed directly without using cartilage as a template?
   a. Intraosseous
   b. Intramembranous
   c. Endochondral
   d. Endosteum
   e. Periosteum

2. Haematoxylin and eosin (H&E) stains blue with which of the following structure?
   a. Nucleus
   b. Erythrocytes
   c. Mitochondria
   d. Cytoplasm
   e. Basophils

3. Which type of epithelium is characteristically associated with goblet cells?
   a. Simple squamous epithelium
   b. Simple cuboidal epithelium
   c. Pseudostratified columnar epithelium

d. Simple columnar epithelium

e. Transitional epithelium

4. Which of the following embryonic structure is the precursor to the greater omentum?

a. Dorsal mesocolon

b. Dorsal mesogastrium

c. Ventral mesentery

d. Dorsal mesoduodenum

e. None of the above

5. Which vessel possesses a characteristic internal and external elastic lamina under a microscopy?

a. Elastic artery

b. Capillaries

c. Arterioles

d. Muscular artery

e. Venules

6. Keratohyalin is a protein found in which layer of the epidermis?

a. Stratum lucidum

b. Stratum corneum

c. Stratum spinosum

d. Stratum basale

e. Stratum granulosum

7. The villi of the small intestine contains which lymphatic capillary structure?

a. Crypt of Lieberkuhn

b. Plicae circulares

c. Lacteal

d. Brunner's glands

e. Peyer's patches

EMQ

For each of the following questions, select the most appropriate answer.

Each option may be used once, more than once or not at all.

A. Type I pneumocyte

B. Macrophage

C. Goblet cells

D. Type II pneumocyte

E. Ciliated cuboidal cells

F. Red blood cells

G. Brush cells

H. Villi

I. Basal cells

J. Clara cells

8. Which cell is considered a squamous alveolar cell?

9. Which cells secrete protein to protect the lining of bronchioles?

10. A baby born at 34 weeks presents with tachypnoea, cyanosis, and subcostal and intercostal retractions. A diagnosis of infant respiratory distress syndrome is made. Which cells are associated with the pathophysiology of this condition?

Chapter 3

METABOLISM

1. A 54-year-old male with a background of anaemia presents to your clinic complaining of feeling tired, and has recently been getting up at night to urinate, three to four times a week. His physical exam is normal, but he has a BMI of 30.
   a. State the normal fasting blood glucose level (1)
   b. State the minimum glucose level for a diagnosis of diabetes in: (1)
      i. Fasting
      ii. Two hours after oral glucose tolerance test
   c. Describe four ways how insulin affects glucose metabolism (4)
   d. Insulin acts as a competitive inhibitor of substrate uridine diphosphate glucose (UDP-glucose). Draw the curve to represent glycogen activity with and without insulin with the x-axis being UDP-glucose and the y-axis being glycogen synthase activity (1)
   e. The HbA1c test is a way to identify plasma glucose control over a prolonged period. Briefly explain the principle behind this test and why it is limited to an average over three months (2)
   f. In this particular patient, which blood test could you request to monitor his blood sugar levels? (1)

2. A 32-year-old presents to your follow-up clinic with test results indicating a total cholesterol level of 8.0 mmol/L (desirable <5.2 mmol/L) and a LDL of 5.5 mmol/L (desirable <2.6 mmol/L). Further tests show evidence of an LDL receptor mutation. A diagnosis of familial hypercholesterolemia is made.
   a. Name a clinical sign of hypercholesterolemia (1)
   b. Give two complications associated with familial hypercholesterolemia (2)
   c. How does cholesterol control cell membrane fluidity and how is this of benefit? (2)
   d. Other than in cell membranes, give two uses of cholesterol in the body (2)
   e. Describe how cells take up LDL (3)

3. A 39-year-old woman complains of lethargy and progressive weight gain despite a decreased appetite. On examination you notice her dry coarse skin, cold peripheries, a pulse of 52 bpm and a goitre. Investigations showed her TSH was 10.0 mU/ml (normal range 0.40–4.0 mU/ml) and her free T4 was 3.5 pmol/L (normal range 9.0–25.0 pmol/L)
   a. Explain the above investigation results and state the diagnosis (3)
   b. What is the most common cause worldwide for this condition? (1)
   c. Explain why the thyroid gland is enlarged (2)

    d. Where is thyroglobulin cleaved by protease enzyme? (1)

    e. Explain why T4 is given as thyroxine replacement and not T3 (1)

    f. Label where T3 and T4 are stored and the follicular cells (2)

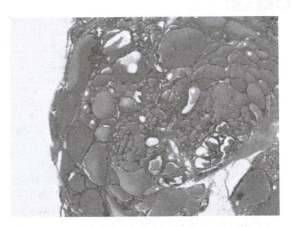

4. Tim, a 19-year-old student, went to see his GP concerned that he had gained a lot of weight since starting university, and that his clothes no longer fitted. The practice nurse was asked to take a dietary history from Tim. She discovered that Tim took very little exercise and that his average daily intake was 16,000 kJ, made up mainly from fast-food and beer.

    a. Name six chemical components of a healthy diet and outline their roles (3)

    b. What is the daily average energy expenditure of a healthy 70 kg adult male? (1)

    c. What three broad components make up the daily energy expenditure of an adult? (2)

    d. Explain in biochemical terms, why Tim has gained weight since coming to university (1)

    e. The student reduces his diet and begins to exercise, yet does not notice any significant reduction in his weight. Why are the results not immediate? (1)

    f. Name four conditions in which being overweight is a risk factor (2)

5. A 40-year-old man is admitted to A&E in an unconscious state. He has a history of alcohol abuse, and you suspect this is a case of alcohol-induced hypoglycaemia.

    a. Explain how alcohol causes hypoglycaemia, and why consuming excessive alcohol cause damage to the liver (2)

    b. Define Km. In this patient, what significance does this have for enzymes in the liver which are responsible for the metabolism of alcohol? (2)

    c. Name two other biochemical changes that are caused by damage to the liver. What symptoms do these present as? (2)

    d. State two symptoms of hypoglycaemia and explain why these occur (2)

    e. Name four community services that are available to the patient (2)

6. A 14-year-old child with type 1 diabetes is admitted to A&E following a collapse whilst playing football.

   Blood tests show the following:
   Blood glucose 14.5 mmol/L, Na 135 mmol/L, K 4.2 mmol/L, Cl 101 mmol/L, bicarbonate 15 mmol/L urea 11.0 mmol/L, creatinine 120 μmol/L, venous pH <7.3, HbA1c 6.2 mmol/L, cortisol 750 nmol/L, β-hydroxybutyrate 1.6 mmol/L, urine and serum ketones +++.

   a. Give two clinical signs that can be seen in this patient (2)
   b. Give approximate volume of urine produced in a 70 kg patient if they have:
      i. Oliguria (1)
      ii. Polyuria (1)
   c. What is β-hydroxybutyrate and why is it high in this patient? (2)
   d. Why is bicarbonate low in this patient? (1)
   e. What are the three hepatic effects of a fall in the insulin:glucagon ratio? (3)

7. A 38-year-old female presents to you complaining of weight gain, fatigue, low mood and muscle weakness. Blood results showed a 9.00 am ACTH 100 ng/L (normal range 0–47 ng/L) and serum cortisol 750 nmol/L (normal range 119–618 nmol/L).
   a. What disorder does this clinical case describe? (1)
   b. Name two other signs or symptoms and briefly explain why they occur (2)
   c. Name two common electrolyte disturbances you would see (1)
   d. Explain why cortisol has a mineralocorticoid effect (1)
   e. Explain the mechanism of how ACTH acts on adrenal cortex (2)
   f. Why in particular is a small-cell carcinoma of the lung likely to secrete ACTH? (3)

8. Patient presents to A&E complaining of right iliac fossa pain, nausea, vomiting and decreased appetite. He has a background of insulin-dependent diabetes.
   a. Describe two macroscopic features of acute appendicitis (2)
   b. Name two microscopic features of an acutely inflamed appendix (2)
   c. This patient has a fever. Which mediators are responsible for producing a febrile response? (1)
   d. Why does polyuria occur in diabetes? (1)
   e. What, if anything, needs to be done to this patient's insulin regimen during his appendicitis and why? (2)
   f. What effect does insulin have on carbohydrate metabolism in the liver and the muscle? (2)

9. A 45-year-old woman presents with increased sweating and palpitations. She has lost around 2 kg in the past six months. She appears agitated and has an obvious non-tender mass on the anterior aspect of her neck.

Her bloods show the following results:
Free T3 of 9.8 pmol/L (normal range 3.5–7.8 pmol/L), free T4 of
48 pmol/L (normal range 9.0–25.0 pmol/L) and TSH of 0.2 mU/L
(normal range 0.40–4.0 mU/L).

a. What is the most likely cause of her thyrotoxicosis? (1)
b. Describe how secretion of the thyroid hormone is controlled (3)
c. What are the effects of the thyroid hormone in humans? (2)
d. What are four anatomical hazards of thyroid surgery? (4)

MCQ

For the following questions, select the single best answer.

1. A 40-year-old woman presents with fever and dysphagia. On examination
   there is a tender and enlarged thyroid gland. Blood tests reveal raised
   T3 and T4 with a decreased TSH. Two months later, the patient returns
   to clinic and is asymptomatic and the thyroid function tests are normal.
   Which of the following is the most likely cause of her presentation?
   a. Hashimoto's thyroiditis
   b. Toxic multinodular goitre
   c. Graves' thyrotoxicosis
   d. De Quervain's thyroiditis
   e. Subacute lymphocytic thyroiditis

2. Which of the following enzymes is stimulated by glucagon?
   a. Acetyl-CoA carboxylase
   b. Glycogen phosphorylase
   c. Glycogen synthase
   d. HMG-CoA reductase
   e. Pyruvate kinase

3. A patient has an insulin-secreting tumour within the pancreas, for which
   she undergoes a 72-hour fast in hospital. What would you expect the test
   results to show?
   a. Proinsulin levels increased
   b. C-peptide levels decreased
   c. Serum glucose levels increased
   d. Glycosylated haemoglobin level increased
   e. Serum insulin levels decreased

4. A 45-year-old man with alcoholic liver disease develops confusion and
   altered level of consciousness. You suspect he has developed hepatic
   encephalopathy where ammonia is not being detoxified. Which amino acid
   typically binds to ammonia to transport and store it in a non-toxic form?
   a. Glycine
   b. Aspartate
   c. Glutamate

d. Lysine
e. Tyrosine

5. A 23-year-old female presents to clinic complaining of shortness of breath and palpitations. On examination you notice she is disproportionately tall and thin with long arms and legs compared to her trunk. On auscultation you hear a systolic murmur. Which protein is affected in this underlying condition?
a. Collagen
b. Crystallin
c. Tau
d. Fibrillin
e. Elastin

6. A lipid analysis from a patient with familial hypercholesterolemia shows elevated LDL and total cholesterol with all other lipid profiles within normal range. Which of the following types of hypercholesterolemia best describes this patient's results?
a. Type Ib
b. Type IIa
c. Type IIb
d. Type V
e. Type III

7. A 58-year-old woman presents with fatigue, feeling cold, with constipation and weight gain. On examination, you notice her skin is dry, she has a pulse rate of 45 beats per minute, and her thyroid is firm and enlarged. Which blood test is likely to confirm the diagnosis?
a. Serum TSH
b. Serum T4
c. Serum T3
d. Anti-thyroid autoantibodies
e. Thyroxin-binding globulin

EMQ

For each of the following questions, select the most appropriate answer.

Each option may be used once, more than once or not at all.

A. Glucose-6-phosphate dehydrogenase
B. Pyruvate dehydrogenase deficiency
C. Phenylketonuria
D. Nicotinamide adenine dinucleotide phosphate (NADPH)
E. Galactosaemia
F. Acetyl-CoA
G. Phosphofructokinase-1
H. Homocystinuria
I. Hexokinase
J. Alpha-ketoglutarate

8. An 8-year-old boy presents with sudden increase in body temperature and yellow colouring of skin and mucous membranes. On examination you notice that his spleen is mildly enlarged. Which deficient metabolite is associated with this condition?

9. Which enzyme is responsible for the rate-limiting step in glycolysis?

10. The mother of a patient has noticed that her child has been experiencing recurrent vomiting and noticed frequent temper tantrums. She has also noticed unusual jerking movement in arms and legs and fair skin. What is the likely diagnosis?

Chapter 4

MEMBRANES AND RECEPTORS

1. A 52-year-old female presents to A&E complaining of a tingling sensation in and around the mouth and lips. Routine blood tests show that her calcium is 1.8 mmol/L (normal range 2.12–2.65 mmol/L). She later becomes bradycardic and is treated with atropine.
   a. For each of the following second messengers, cAMP, cGMP, diacylglycerol, and Ca^{2+}, state which protein kinase they interact with to exert their actions (4)
   b. Describe how calcium influx at nerve terminals causes neurotransmitter release at the synapse (2)
   c. By what two mechanisms are neurotransmitters removed from the synaptic cleft? (1)
   d. Which neurotransmitter is released at:
      i. Sweat glands (1)
      ii. Vascular smooth muscle (1)
   e. What is the effect of atropine on both of the above? (1)

2. A 32-year-old male presents to A&E complaining of light-headedness. His observations show a heart rate of 50 bpm and a blood pressure of 90/55 mmHg.
   a. Which neurotransmitter does parasympathetic preganglionic neurons release and which receptor does it stimulate in the heart? (1)
   b. What are the secondary messengers for muscarinic acetylcholine receptor M_3 and what are their actions? (3)
   c. Draw the electrical conduction graph of the sinoatrial node and label the channels at each point along with their actions (4)
   d. The sinoatrial node generates action potentials at a rate of approximately 100 bpm, but at rest, we have a heart rate of about 60–80 bpm. Why is this? (1)
   e. Which five elements, in order, comprise the cardiac conduction system? (1)

3. A 44-year-old man presents to his doctor complaining of low mood, hallucinations and insomnia. On further questioning you find out he has been drinking around 40 units of alcohol per week for the past 10 years.
   a. Describe how hepatocytes contribute to the pathogenesis of liver cirrhosis in chronic alcoholism (2)
   b. Explain how disulfiram is used to treat chronic alcoholism (1)
   c. Which two common enzymes are responsible for the metabolism of alcohol? (1)
   d. Give two factors that affect drug metabolism in the population (2)

e. Indicate which drug from the graph below has the highest potency, and which drug has the lowest efficacy (1)

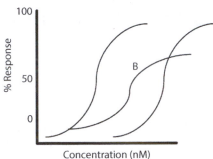

f. Explain why occasionally there is no full response to a drug despite all receptors being occupied (1)

g. What is non-linear kinetics and why is it a problem when consuming alcohol? (2)

4. A 25-year-old female presents with recurrent abdominal pain and fatigue. On examination you notice she is mildly pale with jaundice. The spleen was palpable 5 cm below the left costal margin.

a. Hereditary spherocytosis is often caused by a reduced expression of spectrin. Describe the normal structure of the red blood cell cytoskeleton (2)

b. A blood film shows spherocytes, small round cells. What is the normal shape of a red blood cell? (1)

c. The enzyme LDH was found to be elevated in the plasma. This enzyme is released from red cells. Suggest two conditions affecting other organs that could cause a rise in plasma LDH (1)

d. In anaerobic skeletal muscle what is the function of this enzyme? What happens to the product of the reaction in the tissue? (2)

e. Raised plasma LDH activity is used to monitor the rate of haemolysis. Suggest another biochemical marker that could be used (1)

f. Blood film analysis showed the presence of increased reticulocytes. Explain this observation (1)

g. What would you expect the symptoms of this patient to be? (2)

5. A 30-year-old female presents in your clinic complaining of double vision, periods of blurred vision and distorted colour vision in the left eye for the past few weeks. Recently she has been experiencing bladder problems and loss of coordination manifested by shaky hands, loss of balance and extreme weakness after periods of exercise.

Cerebrospinal fluid showed oligoclonal bands of IgG on electrophoresis. A diagnosis of multiple sclerosis (MS) was confirmed.

a. Which structure in normal nerves becomes damaged in MS? (1)

b. What is the consequence of damage to this structure on nerve conduction velocity? (3)

   c. State what you would expect from the results of a visual evoked
      potential test (1)

   d. Draw a diagram to illustrate the relationship between membrane potential
      and time of an action potential (2)

   e. Describe the stages of an action potential (3)

6. A 55-year-old male presents with shortness of breath, fever and a
persistent productive cough. On examination his heart rate was 110 bpm,
oxygen saturations 90% on room air and there was evidence of bilateral
crackles on auscultation. Community acquired pneumonia (CAP) was
diagnosed.

   a. Name an atypical bacteria that can cause CAP (1)

   b. Looking at this diagram complete the following table (4)

Synapse	Neurotransmitter	Receptor
a		
b		
c		
d		

   c. Indicate three main effects of parasympathetic innervations on the
      lungs (3)

   d. Name the second messenger involved in the parasympathetic and
      sympathetic stimulation in the airways (2)

MCQ

For the following questions, select the single best answer.

1. What is the resting membrane potential for cardiac muscle?
   a. −50 to −70 mV
   b. −20 to −30 mV
   c. −55 to −60 mV
   d. −80 to −90 mV
   e. −90 to −100 mV

2. Which of the following is an example of an extracellular ligand-gated ion channel?
   a. Renal outer medullary potassium channel (ROMK)
   b. Ryanodine receptor
   c. L-type calcium channel
   d. Epithelial sodium channel
   e. Voltage proton channel

3. Which of the following is not a ligand for tyrosine kinase receptors?
   a. Insulin
   b. Epidermal growth factor
   c. GABA
   d. Vascular endothelial growth factor
   e. All of the above

4. Oxaloacetate is an inhibitor of succinate dehydrogenase. What type of enzyme inhibition does this represent?
   a. Competitive
   b. Uncompetitive
   c. Noncompetitive
   d. Irreversible
   e. Allosteric

5. A 35-year-old female presents with muscle weakness. She complains of double vision and drooping of the eye. She describes the weakness being worse during exertion but improves with rest. What is the pathophysiology of this condition?
   a. Antibodies against presynaptic voltage-gated calcium channels
   b. Immune-mediated inflammatory disease against myelinated axons
   c. Antibodies against nicotinic acetylcholine receptors at presynaptic neuromuscular junction
   d. Inflammation of the cavernous sinus and superior orbital fissure
   e. Antibodies against nicotinic acetylcholine receptors at postsynaptic neuromuscular junction

6. Which of the following nerves carry parasympathetic fibres?
   a. Greater splanchnic nerve
   b. Pelvic splanchnic nerves
   c. Lumbar splanchnic nerves
   d. Lesser splanchnic nerves
   e. Sacral splanchnic nerves

7. Which of the following statement describes phase II drug metabolism?
   a. Involves oxidation by cytochrome P-450
   b. Does not include acetylation
   c. Involves conversion to inactive metabolites
   d. Decreases water solubility
   e. All of the above

EMQ

For each of the following questions, select the most appropriate answer.

Each option may be used once, more than once or not at all.

A. cAMP
B. Ca^{2+}
C. cGMP
D. Diacylglycerol (DAG)
E. Protein kinase A (PKA)
F. Nitric oxide
G. Inositol trisphosphate (IP3)
H. Protein kinase C (PKC)
I. Arachidonic acid
J. Calmodulin

8. Which second messenger acts as a signal to release calcium from intracellular stores?

9. Is this only activated in the presence of cAMP?

10. Besides PKA, which other protein is involved in the activation of glycogen phosphorylase?

Chapter 5

MECHANISM OF PATHOLOGY

1. A 48-year-old male presented with painless lymphadenopathy in the neck, groin and axillary lymph nodes. He has no weight loss, cough or night sweats, but has complained of being 'run down' for the past few weeks. Fine-needle aspiration cytology showed reactive follicular hyperplasia.
   a. What is hyperplasia? (1)
   b. Other than as a result of primary malignant neoplasms and metastatic tumour deposits, what are the two most common generic causes of a reactive change in lymph nodes? (1)
   c. What is lymphoma? State the two main categories of lymphomas (2)
   d. Define apoptosis and necrosis. What are the basic differences between the two? (4)
   e. What do you understand by the term staging? State two elements which staging is based on (2)

2. You insert a cannula into a patient to allow them to have IV antibiotics for severe sepsis secondary to pneumonia. The nurses notify you the next day that the arm appears red and swollen around the cannula site.
   a. Name four characteristics of acute inflammation (2)
   b. Name two inflammatory mediators and their functions (2)
   c. Explain the mechanism for the development of hypotension in septic shock (2)
   d. Name two criteria for a diagnosis of systemic inflammatory response syndrome (1)
   e. In septic shock, an infective organism, usually gram-negative bacteria, is implicated. With the aid of a diagram, explain the basis of gram staining (3)

3. A 65-year-old female presents with rectal bleeding and recent change in bowel habit. She complains of unintentional weight loss of around 5 kg in the past 2 months. You suspect she has colorectal carcinoma and send her for an urgent referral.
   a. Name three differences between a benign and a malignant neoplasm (3)
   b. Why might a cancer of the sigmoid colon present earlier than a cancer of ascending colon? (1)
   c. Name two categories of oncogenes that might play a significant role in the development of cancer, and give an example of each gene (2)
   d. Name two extrinsic factors that may play a significant role in the development of cancer (be precise) (2)
   e. Briefly describe the UK bowel cancer screening programme (2)

4. A 22-year-old male has just been involved in a road traffic accident. He has been sent to A&E with an open fracture wound.
   a. Briefly describe the stages involved in fracture healing (2)
   b. Name two differences between first intention and second intention healing (2)
   c. Besides white blood cells, name two cells of granulation tissue (1)
   d. Patient had successful surgery but has been immobile for several weeks and develops a deep vein thrombosis. Briefly describe the processes that result in venous thrombosis (2)
   e. Name one local and one systemic factor that affect wound healing (1)
   f. Anticoagulants are typically used to treat deep vein thrombosis. Describe the difference between low molecular weight heparin (LMWH) and unfractionated heparin (UFH) (2)

MCQ

For the following questions, select the single best answer.

1. A 42-year-old male complains of severe epigastric pain that radiates to the back, fever and nausea, and vomiting. A CT abdomen scan shows an enlargement of the pancreas and peripancreatic collections. Which cellular change is likely to be happening?
   a. Liquefactive necrosis
   b. Coagulative necrosis
   c. Fat necrosis
   d. Caseous necrosis
   e. Wet gangrene

2. A 55-year-old male presents with dysphagia and long-standing burning sensation in the central chest. A gastroscopy is performed and reveals a red appearance of the lower oesophagus with histology showing columnar epithelium with goblet cells. Which process explains this finding?
   a. Hyperplasia
   b. Metaplasia
   c. Neoplasia
   d. Anaplasia
   e. Dysplasia

3. Atherosclerosis is a disease that involves the build-up of plaques inside arteries. These plaques are composed of atheroma, cholesterol crystals and calcification. What is the first visible appearance of atheroma formation?
   a. Ulceration
   b. Thrombus
   c. Collagen
   d. Foam cells
   e. Fatty streak

4. A 21-year-male had an appendectomy 2 months ago. The incision site that was sutured shows localised erythema, induration and pigment alteration. Which cell type is responsible for this inflammatory response?
   a. Giant cell
   b. Eosinophil
   c. Monocyte
   d. Mast cell
   e. Basophil

5. Which finding under microscopy is the best indicator that a tumour is malignant?
   a. Increased nuclear-cytoplasmic ratio
   b. Invasion
   c. Pleomorphism
   d. Giant cells
   e. Normal mitosis

6. A 52-year-old woman presents with fever, chills, night sweats and a productive cough. A sputum suture is positive for acid-fast bacilli and a chest X-ray reveals a right upper lobe cavity with associated consolidation. Which cell is responsible for this lung lesion?
   a. Neutrophil
   b. Natural killer cells
   c. Eosinophil
   d. Erythrocyte
   e. Macrophage

7. Which part of the cell cycle is most sensitive to radiation for the treatment of cancer?
   a. G_0/G_1
   b. G_1/S
   c. S/G_2
   d. G_2/M
   e. M/G_0

EMQ

For each of the following questions, select the most appropriate answer.

Each option may be used once, more than once or not at all.

A. Apoptosis
B. Glutathione
C. Cell swelling
D. Lipase
E. Uric acid
F. Hyaline deposition
G. Free radicals

H. Phagocytosis
I. Haemosiderin deposition
J. Liquefactive necrosis

8. A 16-year-old male was playing in a football match and sustained an injury to his knee. There is an obvious bruise to the area but days later which breakdown product would appear?

9. A 51-year-old female is admitted into hospital following a stroke. She received thrombolytic treatment but sustained cerebral oedema as a result of reperfusion injury. The action of which substance is responsible for this?

10. A 48-year-old male was admitted to A&E following a myocardial infarction. As a result there was myocardial cell death and ischaemic injury to the heart. What appearance would you expect to see under a microscope?

Chapter 6

INFECTION AND IMMUNITY

1. A 10-year-old boy presents with recurrent infections. His blood results reveal absent IgA, and IgG and IgE are both low. He is diagnosed with Bruton's disease.
   a. What is Bruton's disease? (1)
   b. What causes this condition? (1)
   c. What is the long-lasting treatment? (1)
   d. What are the two ways that immunisation can be achieved? (1)
   e. Give one disease example for each of the immunisations you mentioned above that it protects from (1)
   f. Why is the patient asymptomatic for the first three months of his life? (1)
   g. Name four other conditions that are characterised by primary antibody deficiency (4)

2. A 45-year-old male presents to A&E with haemoptysis. He has been experiencing fever, chills and night sweats. He is diagnosed with tuberculosis.
   a. Name two other common causes of haemoptysis (2)
   b. Label the tuberculosis granuloma diagram with the following: giant cells, caseous necrosis, lymphocytes, epithelioid histiocytes (2)

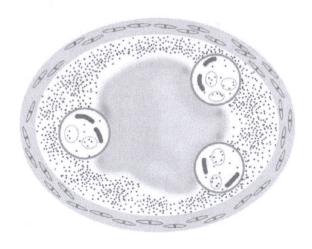

c. Label B7, CD28, MHC class II, CD2, CD4 and TCR on the following T-cell activation diagram (6)

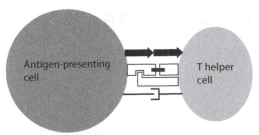

3. A 32-year-old female presents to you with a history of recurrent respiratory infections for the past six months. There have been two occasions that have resulted in hospital admissions. You suspect this patient has humoral immune deficiency.
   a. List three causes of secondary antibody deficiency (1)
   b. Describe three mechanisms of how antibodies work (3)
   c. Draw a diagram explaining the structure of an immunoglobulin antibody (3)
   d. Name two bacterial organisms that can cause infective endocarditis and state what would you look for in the history (3)

4. A 14-year-old girl presents to A&E with difficulty in breathing after developing an acute allergic reaction from a bee sting.
   a. Which antibody is responsible for anaphylaxis and which cells release this? (1)
   b. Briefly explain the pathophysiology of an anaphylactic reaction (4)
   c. Name three reasons for her difficulty in breathing (3)
   d. Explain why she was given adrenaline and corticosteroids (2)

5. A 21-year-old male presents with fatigue and a sore throat for the past week. On examination there is enlarged cervical lymph nodes and tonsils. You suspect tonsillitis and therefore treat with ampicillin. A peripheral blood smear showed lymphocytosis and atypical mononuclear cells.
   a. What are lymphocytosis and atypical mononuclear cells, and what diagnosis is indicated from these findings? (3)
   b. What infective agent is most likely? (1)
   c. Which class of antibody is present? (1)
   d. Why is ampicillin not given to patients with this condition? (1)
   e. State one abdominal sign associated with this condition-how would you detect it? (2)
   f. In a viral infection, which cells are responsible for antigen recognition and how are the antigens generated within a cell? (2)

6. A 14-year-old male presents to you with neck stiffness and photophobia. There are no septic signs and you suspect he has bacterial meningitis.
   a. Haemophilus influenzae is a normal commensal of which area? (1)

b. Name two other causes of bacterial meningitis (1)
c. Name the micro-organism that is stained with:
   i. India ink (1)
   ii. Acid-fast stain (1)
d. What drug would be the best choice for this patient? (1)
e. Explain why this patient is photophobic (1)
f. Name one sign that you can elicit on physical examination which can be a feature of meningitis (1)
g. Label the three layers of the meninges on the following picture (3)

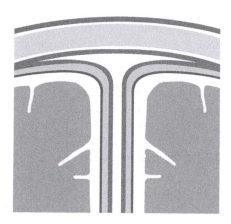

7. A 52-year-old female with a background of diabetes presents to the GP complaining of a two day history of fever, runny nose and a headache. You suspect she has flu.
   a. Which specific influenza virus is the most likely cause? (1)
   b. Which drug would you use to treat her and what is the mechanism of action? (2)
   c. What is the difference between active and passive immunisation? (2)
   d. Name three scheduled immunisations for infants aged 1–6 months in the UK besides hepatitis B (3)
   e. What type of vaccine is hepatitis B? (1)
   f. Name two other blood-borne viruses that are sexually transmitted (1)

MCQ

For the following questions, select the single best answer.

1. Which of the following is an opsonin in the complement system?
   a. C3b
   b. Factor B
   c. C6
   d. Factor H
   e. C5a

2. A 4-year-old boy presents to clinic with a 3-day history of diarrhoea but has only noticed passing blood from the rectum this morning. His blood results reveal a haemoglobin of 98, urea of 12.5 and a creatinine of 110. A blood film examination shows fragmented red cells. Which bacterial infection is likely to cause this presentation?
   a. Salmonella
   b. Campylobacter
   c. Shigella
   d. Staphylococcus
   e. Yersinia

3. A 28-year-old with blood group type A receives a heart transplant from a blood type AB donor. During surgery, after transplantation, the heart was cyanotic, oedematous and mottled. Which of the following statement is the likely explanation?
   a. Acute rejection due to cell-mediated response
   b. Acute rejection due to humoral immune response
   c. Hyperacute rejection due to cell-mediated response
   d. Hyperacute rejection due to preformed ABO blood group antibodies
   e. Chronic rejection due to humoral and cell-mediated response

4. A 57-year-old woman who returned from South America 2 months ago presents to you with productive cough, chest pain and occasional haemoptysis. Sputum culture is positive for acid-fast bacilli. Which principal immune response to this infection will occur?
   a. IgE hypersensitivity
   b. Cell-mediated immunity
   c. Antibody-mediated immunity
   d. Natural killer cell cytotoxicity
   e. Eosinophil-mediated killing

5. A 60-year-old male presents to your clinic with swollen glands in the neck and groin. You suspect a diagnosis of lymphoma and run a test for immunophenotyping. Which of the following cell surface markers are used to identify B cells?
   a. CD3
   b. CD25
   c. CD8
   d. CD19
   e. CD4

6. A study has just released results demonstrating that under expression of J chains is associated with reduced risk of lymphoma. As a consequence, which immunoglobulin(s) would be affected?
   a. IgG
   b. IgA and IgM
   c. IgM
   d. IgE and IgA
   e. IgE

7. Once natural killer cells are activated, which of the following substance is NOT produced?
   a. TNF-alpha
   b. IL-22
   c. Granulocyte macrophage colony stimulating factor
   d. Perforin
   e. IL-10

EMQ

For each of the following questions, select the most appropriate answer.

Each option may be used once, more than once or not at all.

A. Complementary determining region of heavy chain
B. Fragment crystallisable region (Fc region) of light chain
C. Variable region of heavy chain
D. Constant region of heavy chain
E. Variable regions of light and heavy chains
F. Constant regions of light and heavy chains
G. Antigen-binding site of light and heavy chains
H. Fragment crystallisable region (Fc region) of heavy chain
I. Complementary determining region of light chain
J. Variable region of light chain

8. Which determines allotypes?

9. Which determines the antibody's class effect?

10. Which area of the antibody is responsible for opsonisation?

Chapter 7

GASTROINTESTINAL SYSTEM

1. A 35-year-old man presents to A&E following three episodes of vomiting blood. He is known to have oesophageal varices as a result of his alcoholic liver disease.
   a. Define portosystemic anastomosis (1)
   b. Name two other portosystemic anastomoses (2)
   c. Explain the process by which this patient developed oesophageal varices (3)
   d. Given that this is the first time he has vomited, what would happen to the haematocrit level and why? (2)
   e. The patient is given IV isotonic saline solution. How would this affect his intracellular fluid level? Explain why (2)

2. An 18-year-old student presents to your clinic complaining of severe diarrhoea with about 15 bowel movements per day. She describes the motion as oily and extremely foul-smelling. A diagnosis of Crohn's disease is confirmed.
   a. Describe the differences in histology of the duodenum, jejunum and ileum (3)
   b. Explain how damage to the terminal ileum causes steatorrhoea (2)
   c. Explain why the patient may experience macrocytosis (2)
   d. Define jaundice and explain the pathophysiology of pre-hepatic jaundice (3)

3. A 45-year-old construction worker comes to your clinic after noticing a bulge around his groin area. He tells you there is discomfort when he is lifting and he is able to push it back in.
   a. Give two structural features of indirect inguinal hernias (2)
   b. Define hiatus hernia (1)
   c. In a direct hernia, give the three fascial coverings of the hernial sac and say what structures they are derived from (3)
   d. What is meant by physiological herniation? (2)
   e. Through what mechanism are herniations prevented from occurring? (2)

4. A 35-year-old female presents to your clinic complaining with three weeks of epigastric abdominal pain. She describes it as a burning sensation which is relieved after eating. She has a frequent bloating sensation but denies any loss of weight or swallowing difficulties.
   a. Why do you experience epigastric pain with peptic ulcer disease? (2)
   b. Name two hormones that are involved in acid secretion (1)
   c. List four major complications of peptic ulcers (2)
   d. List four structures that are affected if there is a perforation of the posterior wall of the stomach (2)
   e. Name two classes of medications that may be used in the treatment of peptic ulcers. Describe the mechanism of their action (2)
   f. Peptic ulcers are typically associated with helicobacter pylori. What type of bacteria is this? (1)

5. A 30-year-old female comes to your clinic complaining of watery bloody stools for the past six weeks. She experiences cramp-like left abdominal pain that is relieved after a bowel movement. She also has the feeling of constantly needing to pass stools.
   a. Name two differences seen in endoscopy between Crohn's disease and ulcerative colitis (1)
   b. Name two differences seen in histology between Crohn's disease and ulcerative colitis (1)
   c. Name two skin disorders associated with inflammatory bowel disease (1)
   d. State two physiological effects of removing the ascending colon (2)
   e. List two indications for surgery as a treatment for ulcerative colitis (1)
   f. On the following histological diagram of the colon, label the mucosa, muscularis mucosa, submucosa and crypts of Lieberkühn (4)

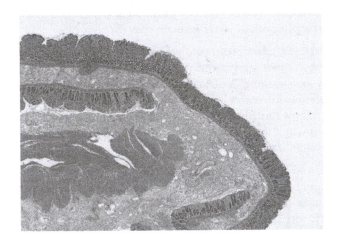

6. A 36-year-old female presents to A&E with right upper quadrant abdominal pain. She has also been experiencing on and off fever and chills for the past week. On examination you notice a yellowish discoloration of her sclera and skin.
   a. What type of jaundice is this? (1)
   b. Explain why a fatty meal can trigger biliary colic (2)
   c. Explain why her stools would be pale and her urine is dark (2)
   d. Briefly describe the recycling of bile (3)
   e. Which enzyme conjugates bilirubin? (1)
   f. Other than pale stools, give another characteristic of stool indicative of jaundice (1)

7. A 40-year-old male presents to you complaining of nausea and vomiting. He has also been experiencing a bloating sensation, epigastric pain and indigestion. He has a history of a duodenal ulcer. A barium swallow studies shows a gastric outlet obstruction.
   a. What is the approximate total daily volume of gastric and bowel secretions? State the types of secretion and their daily volumes (2)

b. What is the possible metabolic status of the patient considering he has been vomiting profusely? Explain how this occurs (2)

c. Explain why a decrease in extracellular fluid volume after vomiting does not trigger the thirst mechanism (2)

d. Describe the muscular layers of the oesophagus (1)

e. Where along the oesophagus are there three normal physiological narrowings? (3)

8. A 42-year-old male presents to A&E with severe epigastric pain radiating to the back. He also complains of nausea and vomiting. He mentions he had a breakdown and consumed two litres of cider after not having alcohol for the past six months.

a. What is the recommended weekly alcohol unit consumption for men and women? (1)

b. What pathological features would you see on microscopy with liver cirrhosis? (1)

c. What disease process could cause his back pain? (1)

d. Which serum enzyme is typically measured for the disease process mentioned? (1)

e. Name two other causes of this disease process (1)

f. Why would this patient have poor vitamin K absorption? (1)

g. The patient recovers but has several more attacks and at an outpatient's appointment his blood glucose is found to be elevated. What has happened? (2)

h. The patient has decided to give up alcohol. Name the stages of the transtheoretical model of behaviour change (2)

9. A 48-year-old female presents to your clinic with upper abdominal discomfort, vomiting and weight loss. She has a reduced appetite which she puts down to having discomfort whilst swallowing. On examination she looks pale and her liver is palpable and enlarged. She is diagnosed with gastric carcinoma.

a. Why does she have poor localised epigastric pain? (1)

b. Label the following on the arterial supply of the stomach (2)

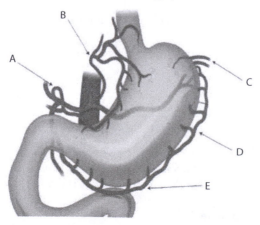

    c. Name two mechanisms the cancer can metastasise other than via the lymphatics (2)

    d. Why does gastric cancer commonly metastasise to the liver? (1)

    e. Name two stimulators of acid secretion from parietal cells. For each stimulator, state the source they are released from (2)

    f. Describe the inhibitory regulation of acid secretion (2)

10. A 50-year-old male presents to your clinic complaining of abdominal pain and weight loss. He describes a heartburn sensation associated with reflux. You suspect he has peptic ulcer disease.

    a. Why does the weight loss suggest this is a gastric ulcer? (1)

    b. The man is suspected of having helicobacter pylori. Explain how these bacteria survive in the acidic condition of the stomach (1)

    c. Name two structures that an ulceration of the posterior wall of the duodenal cap might affect and for one of the structures affected, give the immediate complication (2)

The results of a full blood count from this patient are as follows: Haemoglobin 10 g/L (normal range 130–180 g/L), MCV 65 fL (normal range 80–100 fL), MCH 23 pg (normal range 27–32 pg)

    d. What do the full blood count results suggest/show? (1)

    e. Give an example of the aetiology (1)

    f. Name four parameters you would want to see from the blood results to confirm the diagnosis (2)

    g. What protective mechanism is induced to protect from acid secretion in:

       i. The stomach (1)

       ii. The duodenum (1)

11. A 40-year-old male presents to your clinic with a long history of gastro-oesophageal reflux disease (GORD). He is still complaining of heartburn and now occasional dysphagia. You suspect he has Barrett's oesophagus.

    a. What is the histological name for the change seen in this condition? (1)

    b. What is the epithelial change? (1)

    c. Name the arterial supply of the different portions of the oesophagus (3)

    d. Give four ways in which acid reflux into the lower oesophagus is prevented (4)

    e. What is the nerve supply to the striated muscle in the upper third of the oesophagus? (1)

MCQ

For the following questions, select the single best answer.

1. A 55-year-old obese woman with cirrhosis presents with intermittent severe right upper quadrant pain. She also complains of nausea and vomiting. A diagnosis of gallstones is made. What type of stone is this likely to be composed of?

    a. Cholesterol

    b. Calcium carbonate

   c. Calcium bilirubinate
   d. Cholesterol and calcium carbonate
   e. Calcium oxalate

2. An 8-year-old boy presents with severe diarrhoea and failure to thrive. Enzyme activity from the duodenal juice shows that lipase and amylase are normal but enterokinase is deficient. Which of the following enzymes would be affected as consequence?
   a. Trypsin
   b. Chymotrypsin
   c. Lactase
   d. Elastase
   e. Erepsin

3. The composition of saliva changes upon chewing. Which of the following statements is true regarding the change in stimulated saliva?
   a. Potassium concentration increases
   b. Phosphate concentration increases
   c. Calcium concentration decreases
   d. Flow rate decreases
   e. Sodium concentration increases

4. A 50-year-old woman presents with diarrhoea, bloating and weight loss. She complains that her stools are bulky, foul-smelling, pale and oily. She has tried a gluten-free diet and this has improved. You decide she requires an endoscopy. What would you expect to see from the duodenal biopsy?
   a. Extensive luminal narrowing
   b. Villous atrophy
   c. Crypt abscess
   d. Outpouching of mucosa
   e. Mucosal oedema

5. A 65-year-old man presents with a 4-week history of burning discomfort especially after meals and when lying. An oesophago-gastro duodenoscopy (OGD) shows inflammation of the distal oesophagus. Which of the following best explains this underlying condition?
   a. Helicobacter pylori infection
   b. Absence of oesophageal peristalsis
   c. Protrusion of stomach into thorax
   d. Inappropriate relaxation of lower oesophageal sphincter
   e. Metaplasia of lower oesophagus

6. A patient undergoes an endovascular abdominal aortic aneurysm repair. During the procedure a catheter is inserted into the femoral artery and directed to the aortic aneurysm where the graft extends to the gonadal artery. Which of the following organs is unlikely to lose its blood supply?
   a. Stomach
   b. Diaphragm

c. Descending colon
d. Spleen
e. Adrenal gland

7. A patient undergoes total gastrectomy for gastric cancer. Which of the following vitamin deficiencies would you expect?
   a. Vitamin C deficiency
   b. Vitamin E deficiency
   c. Vitamin B6 deficiency
   d. Vitamin B12 deficiency
   e. Vitamin K deficiency

EMQ

For each of the following questions, select the most appropriate answer.

Each option may be used once, more than once or not at all.

A. Acetylcholine
B. Histamine
C. Gastrin
D. Somatostatin
E. Trypsin
F. Secretin
G. Vasoactive intestinal peptide
H. Sympathetic stimulation
I. Enteroglucagon
J. Vagal cholinergic stimulation

8. Which substance causes secretion of hydrochloric acid and gastrin release from G cells during cephalic phase of gastric acid secretion?

9. Which substance is responsible for the stimulation of bicarbonate secretion in the pancreas?

10. Which substance is released in response to increased serum gastrin levels?

Chapter 8

CARDIOVASCULAR SYSTEM

1. A 63-year-old male comes to your clinic complaining of shortness of breath for the past week, which is particularly worse on lying flat. He fatigues easily and has noticed some weight loss. On examination there is pitting oedema to both lower extremities and inspiratory crackles to the base of both lungs.
   a. In normal circumstances, how is interstitial fluid formed? (2)
   b. Draw a graph comparing a normal heart at rest and heart failure using stroke volume and end diastolic volume as the axes (2)
   c. Explain why patients with heart failure develop oedema (2)
   d. The patient is started on an ACE inhibitor. Explain the effects of this drug on the renal blood flow and glomerular filtration rate (2)
   e. What other class of drug can be given to treat oedema? Please state the mechanism of action (2)

2. A 22-year-old intravenous drug user presents with fever, malaise and a non-productive cough. He is diagnosed with infective endocarditis.
   a. Name the most likely pathogen to cause infective endocarditis in this case (1)
   b. Give one immediate investigation that you would want to perform (1)
   c. Which investigation would you request once he is admitted into hospital? (1)
   d. Name four clinical signs for infective endocarditis during examination (2)
   e. Name four complications of infective endocarditis (2)
   f. The causative organism in this case has a virulence factor that can act as a super antigen. Name the virulent factor (1)
   g. Name another organism that can also act as superantigen (1)
   h. How can this organism's superantigen lead to toxic shock syndrome? (1)

3. The parents of a 6-month-old child are concerned as they describe her being restless and agitated. They have also noticed that the child is sometimes blue in appearance. A diagnosis of tetralogy of fallot (TOF) is confirmed.
   a. Explain the cause of TOF (1)
   b. Give the four typical features of TOF (2)
   c. Explain why the child presented with cyanosis (1)
   d. Label on the following diagram where:
      i. The pulmonary artery and aorta are derived from (1)
      ii. The ventricles are derived from (1)

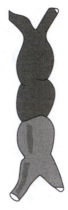

e. What does caudocephalic and lateral folding achieve? (2)
f. Name two other right to left shunt congenital heart defects (2)

4. A 68-year-old male presents for a routine check-up and his BP was found to be 180/90 mmHg. On questioning he has been asymptomatic and is diagnosed with isolated systolic hypertension.
    a. Why do patients acquire left ventricular hypertrophy in hypertension? (1)
    b. What is the anatomical location of the apex beat? (1)
    c. Name two signs associated with left ventricular hypertrophy that can be detected on examination (2)
    d. List three features that stimulate the release of renin (3)
    e. What is the function of renin? (1)
    f. Name two drugs that cause direct acting vasodilation (2)

5. A 55-year-old-woman presents to your clinic complaining of central chest tightness. She reports that the pain occurred while she was running but was relieved upon rest. A diagnosis of stable angina was made.
    a. Which immediate test would you perform? (1)
    b. What abnormality may see expect from this investigation? (1)
    c. This patient is initiated on nitrates. What is the active substance these drugs produce and what is the effect? (2)

The patient returns to your clinic complaining of syncope and shortness of breath and is diagnosed with aortic stenosis.

    d. What type of murmur is associated with this condition? Explain the normal mechanism of aortic valve closure (2)
    e. Which heart sound is heard when the aortic valve is closed? (1)
    f. For each of the valves, indicate the chest surface marking for auscultation:
        i. Mitral (1)
        ii. Pulmonary (1)
    g. What is the role of the National Institute for Health and Care Excellence (NICE) before treatment is available at NHS hospitals? (1)

6. A 28-year-old female has just given birth to her second child. While in hospital she has developed calf pain and tenderness to her right leg. You notice there is swelling, erythema and pitting oedema up to her right knee. A below-knee DVT has been diagnosed.
   a. Name all the blood vessels this thrombus would pass through to get to the lung from the left upper femoral vein (2)
   b. What is ventilation perfusion matching and how is this altered in a pulmonary embolism (PE)? (2)
   c. What is the common finding on an ECG in PE? (1)
   d. With regards to a small pulmonary embolism, which disturbance in acid-base balance would result and why? (2)
   e. This patient was started on warfarin for her DVT. Explain the mechanism of action of this drug, the INR range recommended for a DVT and the duration of anticoagulation in this patient (3)

7. A 70-year-old male presents to your clinic complaining of pain in both his calves after prolonged walking. The pain increases to a point where he has to stop walking, then the pain subsides. He is an ex-smoker and has diabetes. He is diagnosed with peripheral vascular disease.
   a. Explain why the patient experiences pain in the calves (1)
   b. What is the name given to describe this type of pain? (1)
   c. Name two other risk factors of peripheral vascular disease (1)
   d. Which imaging would you perform first to identify the problem in the legs? (1)
   e. Name the pulses of the lower limb, describe their anatomical position and state which pulse is likely to be absent in this case (6)

8. A 63-year-old male presents to your clinic complaining of dizziness, chest pain, syncope and shortness of breath. A diagnosis of aortic stenosis is made.
   a. Explain why in aortic stenosis there is a slow-rising pulse (1)
   b. Explain how aortic stenosis causes chest pain and syncope (2)
   c. Name two causes of aortic stenosis (1)
   d. What is the murmur that is associated with aortic stenosis and how does it arise? (2)
   e. Describe the process of cardiomyocyte contraction (3)
   f. State the main mechanism of intracellular calcium clearance (1)

9. A 3-month-old child presents with feeding difficulties and poor growth. A diagnosis of patent ductus arteriosus (PDA) is made.
   a. What type of murmur would you hear on physical examination? (1)
   b. Briefly describe the direction of blood flow that occurs in PDA and explain why this happens (2)
   c. Name two other foetal shunts that exist and describe their function (4)
   d. Which aortic arch is ductus arteriosus derived from? (1)
   e. Name two other left to right shunt congenital heart defects (2)

10. A 55-year-old male presents to your clinic complaining of palpitations, extreme shortness of breath and coughing up pink stained frothy sputum. Apart for a past history of rheumatic fever as a child, he has no other medical conditions.
    a. Which bacteria typically causes rheumatic fever? (1)
    b. Explain the reason for his deterioration (1)

On further questioning, he says that for the last few days he has been waking in the night because of his breathing and has not been able to sleep lying flat.

    c. What is the mechanism for these symptoms? (2)
    d. His pulse feels irregularly irregular. Name one common cause for this; what one finding on ECG would confirm this diagnosis? (2)
    e. You find that his JVP is raised 7 cm above the reference point. What is used as the reference point and what is the significance of this finding? (2)

After 2 weeks of treatment with diuretics and ACE inhibitor he is seen by his GP. It becomes apparent that he is frustrated and depressed about how long his recovery is taking.

    f. Why is it important that psychological problems in the physically unwell are recognised and treated? (2)

MCQ

For the following questions, select the single best answer.

1. A 28-year-old man presents with a fever and nodules on his finger pads. Blood cultures have shown growth of *Staphylococcus aureus* and an echocardiogram shows the presence of a tricuspid valve vegetation and regurgitation. Which of the following is the likely cause of this condition?
   a. Rheumatic fever
   b. Diabetes mellitus
   c. Congenital heart disease
   d. Intravenous drug user
   e. Alcohol abuse

2. A 19-year-old man presents to A&E complaining of shortness of breath, chest pain and dizziness. You request a chest X-ray to rule out any underlying infection but you notice rib notching. Which underlying congenital heart disease is responsible for this?
   a. Bicuspid aortic valve
   b. Coarctation of aorta
   c. Atrial septal defect
   d. Tetralogy of fallot
   e. Eisenmenger's syndrome

3. A 72-year-old female with a history of hypertension and diabetes presents with chest pains intermittently for 4 days and increasing shortness of breath. She is haemodynamically unstable and on examination you see mottled skin and distended jugular veins. On auscultation there is a third heart sound and end inspiratory crackles. ECG shows ST segment elevation in leads II, III and avF, and reciprocal ST depression in lead I. Which of the following coronary arteries is the most likely affected?
   a. Left anterior descending coronary artery
   b. Right marginal branch artery
   c. Left anterior descending coronary artery
   d. Right coronary artery
   e. Left circumflex artery

4. Which of the following causes ST elevation?
   a. Prinzmetal's angina
   b. Posterior myocardial infarction
   c. Hypokalaemia
   d. Supraventricular tachycardia
   e. Digoxin toxicity

5. Which of the following statements in regards to B-type natriuretic peptide (BNP) is false?
   a. BNP is primarily produced in the atria and ventricles in response to excessive stretching of cardiomyocytes and induces vasoconstriction
   b. BNP induces natriuresis
   c. BNP decreases circulating levels of aldosterone
   d. Endopeptidase is involved in the metabolism of BNP
   e. None of the above

6. A 58-year-old man presents with acute heart failure and undergoes a right heart catheterisation. In which area would you find the lowest oxygen saturations?
   a. Right atrium
   b. Right ventricle
   c. Inferior vena cava
   d. Superior vena cava
   e. Femoral vein

7. Which of the following is NOT a treatment option for transposition of the great arteries?
   a. Atrial switch operation
   b. Arterial switch operation
   c. Prostaglandin E_1 infusion
   d. Atrial septostomy
   e. None of the above

EMQ

For each of the following questions, select the most appropriate answer.

Each option may be used once, more than once or not at all.

A. Aortic stenosis
B. Aortic regurgitation
C. Mitral stenosis
D. Mitral regurgitation
E. Pulmonary regurgitation
F. Tricuspid stenosis
G. Tricuspid regurgitation
H. Aortic sclerosis
I. Patent ductus arteriosus
J. No murmur

8. A 50-year-old female presents to you complaining of diarrhoea, abdominal pain and feeling wheezy. She also states her face becomes hot and red. A CT scan shows a mass in the small intestine and a single nodule in the liver. Which cardiac abnormality is typically associated with this condition?

9. A 58-year-old man presents with shortness of breath, chest pain and dizziness. On examination you notice a slow-rising pulse with a soft S2 heart sound. You hear a crescendo–decrescendo murmur in the second right intercostal space. Which cardiac abnormality will cause this presentation?

10. A 65-year-old female presents to you with shortness of breath especially when she lies down, and swollen ankles. On examination you notice an irregular pulse and a holosystolic murmur at the apex of the heart that radiates to the axilla. Which cardiac abnormality will cause this presentation?

Chapter 9

RESPIRATORY SYSTEM

1. A 63-year-old ex-smoker comes to your clinic complaining of dry cough and a general feeling of discomfort. He has also been experiencing shortness of breath, especially when exercising. On examination you notice clubbing of his fingers and bibasal inspiratory crepitations. You suspect he has pulmonary fibrosis.
   a. Draw a graph showing the curve for lung compliance in normal and lung fibrosis patients (3)
   b. For the following, indicate whether the pulmonary function test results for this patient would show normal, an increase or decrease.
      i. Total lung capacity (1)
      ii. Residual volume (1)
   c. Explain why patients with lung fibrosis have reduced chest expansion during inspiration (1)
   d. The transfer factor of the lung for carbon monoxide is reduced. What does this result signify? (1)
   e. Name three structural barriers for oxygen to pass from alveolar air to red blood cell/pulmonary capillary blood (3)

2. A 65-year-old female presents with a 4-week history of a non-productive cough and shortness of breath. She has also noticed weight loss and describes hoarseness to her voice. She has a 40 pack-year history.
   a. Why does she have a hoarse voice? (1)
   b. What three mechanisms determine the spread of cancer? (3)
   c. Why is this patient more prone to respiratory infections compared with a healthy 57-year-old man? (1)
   d. What is TNM? What do Tis, N0 and M0 mean? (1)
   e. What is the percentage incidence of each of the main four types of lung cancer? (4)

3. A 58-year-old male presents with worsening dyspnoea and increased sputum production. He feels fatigued and complains his chest sounds wheezy. He is a retired construction worker.
   a. What is the major cause for COPD in the UK? (1)
   b. Name two histological changes that occur in the bronchioles in chronic bronchitis (2)

   Below is an example of this patient's arterial blood gas (ABG) test:
   pH 7.35 (7.35–7.45), PaO_2 7.8 (9.3–13.3 kPa), $PaCO_2$ 8.0 (4.7–6.0 kPa), HCO_3 32 (22–28 mmol/L)

   c. What type of respiratory failure do the results show? (1)
   d. What is the acid base status and why? (2)

    e. Where are the central and peripheral chemoreceptors located? (2)

    f. What is the difference in the response of the central and peripheral chemoreceptors to prolonged hypercapnia and hypoxia? (2)

4. A 15-year-old female is brought into A&E due to an asthma attack. Her respiratory rate is 28 per minute, heart rate is 115 bpm and you notice there is blueness to her fingers, lips and tongue.

    a. What is the name given to this blue discoloration? (1)

    b. Why does the patient have tachycardia? (2)

    c. Name four common causes of hypoxaemia (2)

    d. What are the main structures in the lung that are affected? (1)

    e. Give four histological changes associated with asthma (2)

    f. Name two classes of drugs that you would treat initial stages of asthma with and describe their general mechanism of action (2)

5. A 42-year-old male presents with a persistent cough, chest pain and shortness of breath. A chest X-ray was ordered and shows left sided pleural effusion.

    a. Name two causes of exudative pleural effusion (1)

    b. What is the innervation of the pleura? (2)

    c. The patient undergoes a thoracentesis. Where would you typically insert the needle and why? (2)

    d. What structures does the needle pass through during a thoracentesis to reach the pleural cavity? (2)

    e. Why might a person with pleurisy feel pain in the umbilical region? (1)

    f. What is the innervation to the main muscle used in breathing and what is its nerve root? (2)

6. A 60-year-old male presents complaining of long-term breathlessness and a persistent dry cough. On examination there are fine-end inspiratory crackles. He worked as a heating engineer for over 20 years.

    a. Below is a histology slide of the trachea. Label the following structures: A–D (2)

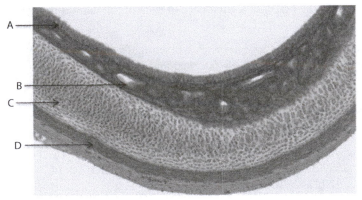

Reproduced with permission of Dr Ana Gonzalez and Prof Giles Perryer

    b. Explain the pathophysiology of asbestosis (1)

c. Infections are a common complication of pulmonary fibrosis. Name three commensal organisms of the upper respiratory tract (1)
d. Explain how PaO_2 and $PaCO_2$ will alter in chronic fibrotic lung disease and how this will affect the acid base balance (1)
g. Explain how acid base disturbance affects oxygen binding in erythrocytes (1)
h. The following is a spirometry volume-time curve. Name the pattern of lung disease indicated by curve X and explain how you derived your answer (2)

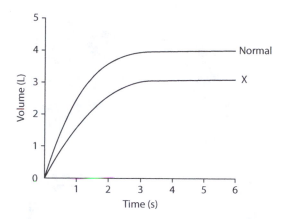

e. Describe the impact of chronic illnesses on an individual's life (2)

7. A 38-year-old female presents with 2-day history of breathlessness, a high fever and coughing up yellow sputum.
    a. Give three mechanisms whereby infections are normally prevented from gaining access to the respiratory tract (3)
    b. You make a diagnosis of left lower lobe consolidation; give two physical signs that would be apparent (2)
    c. Give three common bacterial organisms that can cause community acquired pneumonia (1)
    d. The patient was started on penicillin. What is the mechanism of action of this drug? (1)
    e. Describe three factors which might affect a patient's adherence to the treatment (3)

8. A young girl was involved in a fight injuring the left side of her thorax and she collapsed on the ground. She was struggling to breathe with shallow breathing. On examination you notice tachypnoea, tachycardia, cyanosis and hyper-resonance to percussion, diminished breath sounds on the left side of her thorax and the trachea is deviated to the right.
    a. What is the most likely diagnosis and why? (2)
    b. Explain the difference between peripheral and central cyanosis (2)
    c. What would be your immediate management in this case? (1)
    d. What is the significance of the deviation of the trachea? What might be the consequence of this? (2)

e. What type of joint is a costochondral joint? (1)

f. What are the accessory muscles of inspiration? (2)

9. A 40-year-old male presents to your clinic complaining of shortness of breath and a cough with purulent sputum. He says he is not feeling himself and feels hot at times.

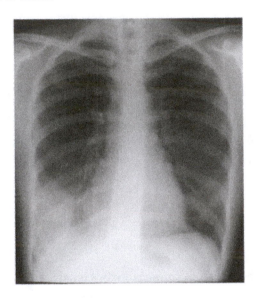

a. From the above chest X-ray, describe what you see (1)

b. Name two things you may hear on auscultation (2)

c. Work out the concentration of HCO_3 from the Henderson–Hasselbach's equation and state what acid base balance this patient is in (3)

His arterial blood gas showed the following: pH 7.25, $PaCO_2$ 66 mmHg, PaO_2 9.0 kPa

$$pH = 6.1 + \log \frac{\left(\left[HCO_3^-\right]\right)}{\left(0.03 \times pCO_2\right)}$$

d. What is the most likely organism to cause this? (1)

e. Which antibiotic is most commonly used to treat this condition? (1)

f. What class of drug would you use if the patient was allergic to the treatment in (e) and what is the mechanism of action? (2)

10. A 45-year-old male presents with a persistent cough that has been ongoing for more than 4 weeks. He mentions that on occasions he has been coughing up blood and has been very short of breath. He has noticed his trousers have become looser. A diagnosis of bronchial adenocarcinoma is made.

a. What is epithelium of the main bronchus? (1)

b. Is this tumour malignant or benign? Define this term (1)

c. Name two nerves which could be damaged around the left hilar region and the associated symptoms from a bronchial carcinoma (2)
d. This patient undergoes a pulmonary function test and results show FVC = 3.2 L and FEV$_1$ = 2.5 L. Comment on this finding (2)
e. Give two tests to differentiate between obstructive and restrictive deficit in this patient (2)
f. The patient's right lower lobe was removed. State the two fissures that divide the right lung and their surface markings (2)

MCQ

For the following questions, select the single best answer.

1. A 25-year-old male presents to A&E after chest trauma. He has been experiencing difficulty in breathing and a chest X-ray and CT scan showed a massive pleural effusion with collapse of the left lung. A chest drain was inserted with a white-yellow fluid flowing out. A diagnosis of thoracic duct rupture was made. In which of the following regions is the thoracic duct located?
   a. Middle and posterior mediastinum
   b. Anterior and middle mediastinum
   c. Superior and posterior mediastinum
   d. Superior and middle mediastinum
   e. Superior and anterior mediastinum

2. A 4-year-old child presents to A&E following an aspirated foreign body. It was witnessed by parents that this was a nut fragment. Where in the bronchi would this typically lodge?
   a. Superior segment of right inferior lobe
   b. Lateral segment of right middle lobe
   c. Apical segment of right superior lobe
   d. Apico-posterior segment of left superior lobe
   e. Superior segment of left inferior lobe

3. A 56-year-old man presents to you complaining of shortness of breath and a productive cough. He has a 30 pack-year smoking history and you suspect he has COPD. You perform a spirometry. Which of the following cannot be measured using this method?
   a. Forced vital capacity
   b. Tidal volume
   c. Vital capacity
   d. Forced expiratory flow
   e. Functional residual capacity

4. A 50-year-old male presents with shortness of breath, chest pain, weakness and leg swelling. On examination there is a loud pulmonary second heart sound, systolic murmur and a raised jugular venous pressure (JVP).

A diagnosis of pulmonary hypertension is made. What would you expect to see on a JVP waveform?
a. Absence of a wave
b. Large a waves
c. Slow y descent
d. Prominent v waves
e. No changes

5. A 60-year-old female presents complaining of a chronic productive cough, shortness of breath and feeling wheezy. She has a significant smoking history and on examination you notice tachypnoea and use of accessory muscles. Which of the following pulmonary function tests best describes a diagnosis of emphysema?
   a. FEV_1/FVC <0.7, Decreased residual volume, Low diffusing capacity of the lung (DLCO)
   b. FEV_1/FVC <0.7, Decreased residual volume, Normal DLCO
   c. FEV_1/FVC >0.7, Decreased residual volume, High DLCO
   d. FEV_1/FVC >0.7, Increased residual volume, Normal DLCO
   e. FEV_1/FVC >0.7, Increased residual volume, Decreased DLCO

6. A 35-year-old female presents with fever, rigors and malaise. She becomes unwell and complains of a pleuritic chest pain and haemoptysis. On examination she is tachycardic and tachypnoea. What other sign on examination would you expect?
   a. Vesicular breath sounds
   b. Decreased vocal resonance
   c. Dull percussion note
   d. Increased chest expansion
   e. Decreased tactile vocal fremitus

7. Which of the following statements with regard to cystic fibrosis is FALSE?
   a. Cystic fibrosis is an autosomal recessive disease.
   b. Cystic fibrosis is associated with mutations in the CF transmembrane conductance regulator (CFTR) gene on chromosome 5.
   c. CFTR is an ATP-responsive chloride channel.
   d. At least 85% of patients with cystic fibrosis have pancreatic insufficiency.
   e. The estimated survival is now between 40 and 50 years old.

EMQ

For each of the following questions, select the most appropriate answer.

Each option may be used once, more than once or not at all.

A. Right sided pneumothorax
B. Left-sided pneumothorax
C. Tension pneumothorax
D. Right sided pleural effusion

E. Left sided pleural effusion
F. Cardiac failure
G. COPD
H. Asthma
I. Bronchiectasis
J. Pulmonary embolus

8. A 55-year-old male presents with sudden shortness of breath and pleuritic chest pain. On examination he is tachypnoea and there is stony dull percussion and reduced chest expansion on the affected side. A chest X-ray shows blunting of the costophrenic angle and the trachea is deviated to the right side. What is the diagnosis?

9. A 40-year-old female presents to A&E with shortness of breath. She looks distressed and is sweating. Her pulse is 140 beats per minute, there is reduced chest expansion and hyper-resonant percussion. A chest X-ray shows the trachea is deviated away from the side of collapse. What is the diagnosis?

10. A 62-year-old smoker presents with shortness of breath, chest pain and haemoptysis. He has been admitted six times to the hospital for chest infections in the past year. On examination there are coarse bilateral crackles at the bases of his lung and large airway rhonchi. You also notice clubbing. What is the diagnosis?

Chapter 10

URINARY SYSTEM

1. A 48-year-old male with a background of diabetes presents to you
   complaining of swelling in his legs and puffiness around his eyes.
   A diagnosis of nephrotic syndrome is made.
   a. Below is a histology picture of a renal parenchyma. Label the
      glomerulus (1)

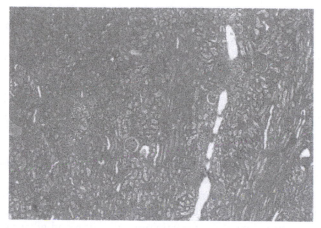

   b. Which cells line the visceral layer of the Bowman's capsule? (1)
   c. Name a type 2 and type 3 hypersensitivity reaction disorder that can
      cause glomerulonephritis (2)
   d. Name three barriers between the glomerulus and the Bowman's
      capsule (3)
   e. Give two reasons why proteins cannot cross the glomerular tuft (2)
   f. This patient is diagnosed with diabetes. What will happen to the
      volume and osmolality of urine after it has passed the proximal
      convoluted tubule? (1)

2. A 52-year-old male with a background of hypertension and coronary heart
   disease presents to A&E with nausea and vomiting. He also complains of
   fatigue and headache. You decide to perform an ABG.
   a. From the ABG results what is the acid-base status of this patient? (1)
      pH 7.20, PaO_2 11.5 kPa, $PaCO_2$ 4.2 kPa, HCO_3 16.5 mmol/L
      Na 140, K 6.5, Cl 99
   b. Calculate the anion gap (1)
   c. Name two causes of the above results (2)
   d. Below is a diagram of the proximal tubule. Annotate the diagram with
      pumps responsible for H^+ secretions (3)

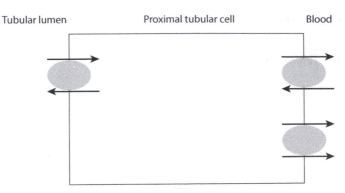

Tubular lumen   Proximal tubular cell   Blood

e. The patient's serum potassium level is high. Give one cause of hyperkalaemia and name a substance that you can administer to stimulate Na^+/K^+-ATPase to bring the potassium back to normal level. Explain the mechanism (3)

3. A 32-year-old male presents to your clinic complaining of blood in his urine. He also experienced pain in the right flank which initially started from the back, accompanied with nausea and vomiting.
   a. What is the anatomical origin of the pain? (1)
   b. The patient undergoes an X-ray of the kidney, ureter and bladder. Explain the course of the ureter on X-ray (3)
   c. A CT scan revealed dilatation of the renal pelvis. Explain how this obstruction can cause a change in the glomerular filtration rate (2)
   d. Where is the primary site for calcium regulation and what are the two transporters responsible for its excretion? (2)
   e. Give two chemical signals that control serum calcium. For each signal, state where they are secreted from (2)

4. A 55-year-old male comes to your clinic for an annual review. On examination his blood pressure measurement was 160/85 mmHg and you hear an epigastric bruit. You suspect he has renal artery stenosis.
   a. Explain how renal artery stenosis would lead to hypertension (2)
   b. What is renin and what does it do? (2)
   c. Explain why this patient might suffer from hyperkalaemia (2)
   d. What would you be able to find in an ultrasound of this man's kidneys? (2)
   e. This patient was started on ACE inhibitor and he returns for a review 1 month later. However, his blood pressure still remains high and his renal function is deteriorating. Explain why this is the case (2)

5. A 70-year-old male presents to you complaining of increased urinary frequency and having to wake up at night at least three times a week to go to the toilet. He has noticed some blood in his urine but has not lost any weight and has a good appetite.
   a. In the diagram below, label the prostate gland, urethra, ureter and vas deferens (2)

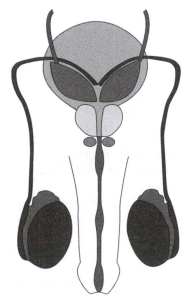

b. The urologist would like to do a cystoscopy. Name the three parts of the urethra that he would have to pass through to reach the prostate (1)

c. Name the anterior, posterior and superior anatomical relations of the prostate (3)

d. Briefly explain the process of micturition and the nerves involved (4)

6. A 62-year-old female with a background of congestive heart failure presents to A&E after falling over at home. She is confused and clinically looks dehydrated.

A series of blood tests were carried out and below are her U&Es results: Na 141, K 4.8, urea 18.5, creatinine 230, eGFR 45.

a. Work out creatinine clearance and comment on the eGFR. (2) Her weight is 55 kg.

$$CrCl = \frac{(140 \ age) \times weight \times 1.04}{Serum \ creatinine}$$

b. How would raised sodium affect urine osmolality? (1)

c. How do cells survive in a high osmotic environment? (1)

d. What hormone is secreted in response? (1)

e. What channel does this hormone work on, and which part of the kidney does it act on? (2)

f. For the following question, select the appropriate volume in a standard 70 kg man.
   i. 35 L
   ii. 350 ml
   iii. 3.5 L
   iv. 42 L

   v. 4.2 L
  vi. 420 ml
 vii. 2.8 L
viii. 280 ml
  ix. 28 L
     I.   Total plasma volume? (1)
    II. Total water in the body? (1)
  III. Total intracellular fluid? (1)

7. A 65-year-old male comes to A&E with difficulty passing urine and describes a sensation of a full bladder that is now causing discomfort.
   a. A transurethral catheter was attempted but failed. What method should be attempted next if access via the urethra was restricted? Explain the anatomical basis (2)
   b. Give two possible findings on physical examination causing this urinary retention (2)
   c. What should be measured in the blood test? (1)
   d. Which nerves and nerve roots are responsible for filling and voiding of the bladder? (3)
   e. This patient was diagnosed with prostatic adenocarcinoma. Label on the diagram below the prostate region where malignancies usually develop, and explain why this is important (2)

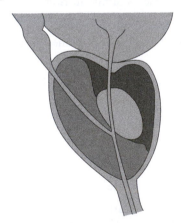

8. A 38-year-old male was on holiday and suddenly developed excruciating spasms in the loin that radiated to the groin. He also complained of nausea and vomiting, dysuria and increased urinary frequency.
   a. Name two parameters that you would attempt to detect in urine microscopy in this patient? (1)
   b. What kind of impairment of the kidney has occurred? (1)
   c. What is normal adult urine output? (1)

d. The patient suddenly becomes dehydrated with associated hyponatraemia and hypokalaemia. Why has this occurred? (1)

e. The doctors cannot decide which imaging technique to use. Describe the difference between intravenous pyelogram and ultrasound imaging of the kidney (1)

f. Name three locations where renal stones are typically deposited (3)

g. This patient is in excruciating pain. What initial analgesia would you start this patient on, and what is the mechanism of action of this drug? (2)

9. A 70-year-old male presents to you complaining of a 1-month history of poor stream, terminal dribbling and hesitancy.

a. Describe the course of the ureters in the male (2)

b. The prostate gland secretes a milky, slightly acidic fluid that contains several important substances. Name two substances and for each, identify its function (2)

c. What are the adult derivatives of Wolffian and Müllerian ducts in the reproductive system? (1)

d. What system is used to grade prostate cancer? (1)

e. Name two features that are used to grade malignancies (1)

f. Explain why prostate cancer may be associated with back pain and how this occurs (3)

MCQ

For the following questions, select the single best answer.

1. A 55-year-old male presents with abdominal pain and is unable to pass urine. On examination his bladder is tender and distended, and a bladder scan shows 750 ml. You decide to catheterise the patient. Where is the first site of resistance encountered on catheter insertion?
   a. Membranous urethra
   b. Urethral meatus
   c. Bulbar urethra
   d. Prostatic urethra
   e. Penile urethra

2. A 43-year-old female complains of flank pain with nausea and vomiting. You decide to do an ultrasound of the kidney, which shows a bright, highly reflective lesion in the left kidney. Which of the following is the most likely cause?
   a. Renal cell carcinoma
   b. Multiple renal cysts
   c. Angiomyolipoma
   d. Renal lymphoma
   e. Renal adenoma

3. A 60-year-old male presents with suprapubic pain, and nausea and vomiting. On examination you detect a distended bladder. Ultrasound of the kidney shows hydronephrosis. Which of the following renal function will NOT be impaired?
   a. Glomerular filtration rate
   b. Renal blood flow
   c. Creatinine
   d. Blood urea nitrogen
   e. Urinary diluting ability

4. A 32-year-old male presents with sudden severe loin pain and haematuria. He complains that the pain moves to the groin. A CT scan reveals kidney stones. Which of the following is NOT an anatomical site where kidney stones typically become lodged?
   a. Ureterovesical junction
   b. Ureteropelvic junction
   c. Calyx of the kidney
   d. Pelvic ureter
   e. Vesical orifice

5. A 65-year-old female presents with renal colic and haematuria. She has also been complaining of polyuria and polydipsia. Clinically she looks dehydrated and fatigued. Blood results show a raised calcium, raised parathyroid hormone (PTH) and raised phosphate. Which of the following statements is true with regards to the function of PTH on the kidneys?
   a. Increases release of calcium
   b. Promotes production of active vitamin D
   c. Increases calcium and phosphate absorption
   d. Decreases calcium and increases phosphate absorption
   e. Increases phosphate absorption

6. Which of the following statements regarding control of the bladder is FALSE?
   a. Sympathetic postganglionic neurons activate β3 adrenergic receptors causing relaxation of bladder smooth muscle
   b. Sympathetic postganglionic neurons activate α-1 adrenergic receptors causing contraction of urethral smooth muscle
   c. Parasympathetic postganglionic neurons stimulate M2 muscarinic receptors causing bladder contraction
   d. Somatic axons in the pudendal nerve activate nicotinic cholinergic receptors causing contraction of external sphincter striated muscle
   e. All the above are FALSE

7. A 62-year-old male presents with high blood pressure that cannot be controlled with medication. Doppler ultrasound of the kidney shows the renal artery diameter to be less than 75%. What effect would you expect?
   a. Decreased glomerular filtration rate (GFR), decreased renal blood flow, no change in filtration fraction

b. Decreased GFR, decreased renal blood flow, increased filtration fraction
c. No change in GFR, decreased renal blood flow, increased filtration fraction
d. Increased GFR, decreased renal blood flow, increased filtration fraction
e. Increased GFR, increased renal blood flow, no change in filtration fraction

EMQ

For each of the following questions, select the most appropriate answer.

Each option may be used once, more than once or not at all.

A. Respiratory acidosis
B. Respiratory alkalosis
C. Metabolic acidosis
D. Metabolic alkalosis
E. Mixed metabolic and respiratory acidosis
F. Mixed metabolic and respiratory alkalosis
G. Respiratory acidosis with metabolic compensation
H. Respiratory alkalosis with metabolic compensation
I. Metabolic acidosis with respiratory compensation
J. Metabolic alkalosis with respiratory compensation

8. A 65-year-old man with a background of chronic obstructive pulmonary disorder is admitted to A&E with a blood pressure of 80/45 mmHg, heart rate of 100 bpm, respiratory rate of 25 and confusion. His blood gas shows a pH 7.15, PaO_2 7.5 kPa, $PaCO_2$ 9.2 mmHg, HCO_3 15 mmol/L. What is the diagnosis?

9. A 47-year-old female presents with muscle weakness and tremor. She is on a thiazide diuretic and her potassium level is 2.2 mmol/L. Her blood gas shows pH 7.52, PaO_2 8.0 kPa, $PaCO_2$ 7.8 mmHg, HCO_3 40 mmol/L. What is the diagnosis?

10. A young girl presents to A&E following an overdose of morphine. Her blood gas shows pH of 7.30, PaO_2 8.0 kPa, $PaCO_2$ 8.0 mmHg, HCO_3 25 mmol/L. What is the diagnosis?

Chapter 11

MUSCULOSKELETAL SYSTEM

1. A 20-year-old female tried committing suicide by cutting the flexor line of her wrist at the palmar surface using razor blade and is bleeding profusely.
   a. Which structures are affected if the radial side of the wrist is cut? (2)
   b. She has lost sensation at the central palmar surface of the hand. Why? (1)
   c. She experiences weakened flexion of the wrist. Which two tendons that are innervated by the median nerve are involved? (2)
   d. However, she retains sensation at the medial one and a half fingers. Why? (1)
   e. Which two groups of intrinsic muscles of the hand are supplied by the same nerve? (2)
   f. When the radial artery is ligated at the wrist, the hands and fingers usually do not suffer from ischaemia; why? (2)

2. A 6-year-old child falls on to an outstretched hand while climbing a tree. He refuses to move the elbow and there is obvious swelling and deformity. An X-ray shows a supracondylar fracture of the humerus.
   a. Which artery is affected with this type of fracture? (1)
   b. How does a haematoma form from this injury? (1)
   c. What four symptoms/signs would there be in loss of blood supply to the forearm? (2)
   d. What cells are osteoblasts and osteoclasts derived from? (1)
   e. Shade in the sensory distribution of the nerve that is most commonly damaged with this fracture and name this nerve (be precise) (2)

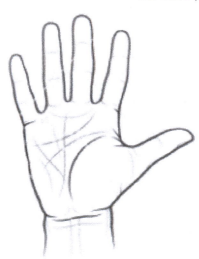

    f. Describe two motor tests you could do to assess the status of this nerve (2)

    g. She was given a cast; after 4 months, why did the bone not heal? (1)

3. A 25-year-old cyclist sustained a clavicle fracture following a fall from his bike. The patient holds the affected arm adducted close to the body, supporting it with the opposite hand. X-rays reveal a mid-shaft clavicle fracture.

    a. A clavicle fracture can occasionally cause secondary injury to the brachial plexus. What is another name for an upper brachial plexus injury, and what nerve roots are affected? (2)

    b. Name two vessels that may be damaged in association with this fracture (2)

    c. How may the lateral and medial ends of the clavicle be displaced as a result of the fracture? Explain your answer (3)

    d. Name two functions of the clavicle (2)

    e. Why is it important to auscultate the chest of this patient? (1)

4. A mother of a 4-year-old child is concerned as she has noticed that her child seems less mobile on one side. On examination you notice an abnormal gait. You suspect this is developmental dysplasia of the hip.

    a. Define a waddling gait (1)

    b. State two non-physical consequences of unresolved congenital hip dysplasia (CHD) in the child (2)

    c. State one physical abnormality of CHD in an adult (1)

    d. Complete the following table: (6)

	Major nerve	Dermatome
Hip flexion		
Leg adduction		
Knee flexion		

5. A rugby player was injured during a game and heard a 'pop' from his shoulder. On examination he is in extreme pain with limited range of movement. X-ray reveals a shoulder dislocation.

    a. Three months after reduction, a contour appears on the shoulder without further dislocation. Why has this contour appeared? (2)

    b. Superior shoulder dislocation is uncommon. Which other joint is involved? (1)

    c. Where do the rotator cuff tendons insert? (1)

    d. Other than rotator cuffs, state two features aiding shoulder stability. (2)

    e. Which muscle is responsible for initial abduction at the shoulder? (1)

    f. Another patient comes to your clinic with right-sided shoulder pain on abduction from approximately 70 degrees – 120 degrees. What is this called? Explain your answer (2)

    g. What is subluxation? (1)

6. A 54-year-old female who works as a secretary comes to your clinic complaining of lower back pain that radiates down the back of her left leg. She also been experiencing pins and needles and numbness in her left leg. She is diagnosed with sciatica.
   a. Name the ligament that runs anteriorly to the vertebrae (1)
   b. Which structure of the intervertebral disc is:
      i Ruptured (1)
      ii. Herniated (1)
   c. Which imaging is best to investigate this type of injury? (1)
   d. MRI shows compression of the L5 nerve. Explain the dermatomal distribution of L5 (1)
   e. Give two muscles that involve dorsiflexion of the ankle (2)
   f. Cervical vertebrae C7 has a much longer spinous process which helps in identifying it as a bony landmark. How else does it differ from the other cervical vertebrae? (1)

   She returns 3 weeks later complaining she has been experiencing problems in controlling her bladder

   g. What is the role of sacral parasympathetic fibres in micturition? (2)

7. A 68-year-old woman sustains a fall on to her right hip while walking the dog. She complains of severe hip pain and is unable to weight bear.
   a. Why are elderly people more prone to falls? Suggest two reasons (2)
   b. Describe how the affected leg would look in a neck of femur fracture (1)
   c. Name the arteries supplying the head of the femur (2)
   d. Hip fractures are usually classified according to anatomy. Explain:
      i. The difference between intra- and extracapsular hip fractures (1)
      ii. The clinical significance in determining whether the patient has intra- or extracapsular hip fracture (1)
   e. What is osteoporosis and why is it more common in elderly women? (2)
   f. Name two adverse consequences of hospitalisation (1)

8. A 70-year-old woman sustains a Colles' fracture of her right wrist.
   a. Describe briefly what type of fall would lead to a Colles' fracture and why? (2)
   b. Give two factors which prejudice the healing of fractures (1)
   c. Name two possible long-term problems that may follow from a Colles' fracture (2)
   d. What is a pathological fracture? (1)
   e. The patient also has some tenderness at the base of her thumb. You suspect a possible scaphoid fracture. What is the commonest site of fracture of the scaphoid? (1)
   f. What imaging method would you order? (1)
   g. What is the complication associated with this type of fracture? Why does this occur? (2)

9. A 35-year-old old man sustained a stab wound to the groin during a fight. There was no damage to the genitalia. He arrives to you alert and orientated but in some distress.
   a. Which superficial vein was damaged? (1)
   b. Describe the sensory loss from the nerve damage in (a) (2)
   c. He is able to dorsiflex his ankle but cannot plantarflex. Which nerve is damaged? State the nerve roots (2)
   d. Label the femoral artery, lateral circumflex artery, external iliac artery and dorsalis pedis artery (2)

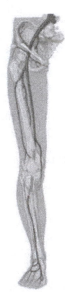

   e. Indicate the superior, medial and lateral borders of the femoral triangle (3)

MCQ

For the following questions, select the single best answer.

1. A 35-year-old male presents with increasing pain affecting the back and buttock area, which radiates to the hip. He has a previous diagnosis of vertebral osteomyelitis. On examination he has a fever, tenderness at the back and right hip pain on hyperextension while lying flat. You also notice a soft swelling on his back and groin area. Which path would you expect the abscess to track to?
   a. Sartorius
   b. Rectus femoris
   c. Psoas major
   d. Gluteus minimus
   e. Vastus lateralis

2. A 42-year-old female with a background of hypothyroidism presents complaining of tingling, pain and numbness in her fingers. She mentions that these symptoms are worse at night. On examination which deficit would you expect?
   a. Loss of sensation over the first web space of the dorsum of the hand
   b. Loss of sensation over the lateral half of the dorsum of third finger
   c. Reduced adduction of the thumb of the affected hand
   d. Reduced extension of the thumb at the metacarpophalangeal joint of the affected hand
   e. Reduced flexion of second and third digits at the metacarpophalangeal joints of the affected hand

3. An 18-year-old male presents to you after an injury to his right shoulder while playing rugby. X-rays show an anterior dislocation of the shoulder joint. Which of the following nerves will most likely be injured as a consequence of this?
   a. Dorsal scapular nerve
   b. Axillary nerve
   c. Long thoracic nerve
   d. Suprascapular nerve
   e. Lower subscapular nerve

4. A 55-year-old male presents complaining of lower back pain and numbness. On examination you notice that during the swing phase of his gait his right pelvis dips below level. Injury to which nerve is responsible for this clinical picture?
   a. Superior gluteal nerve
   b. Inferior gluteal nerve
   c. Femoral nerve
   d. Sciatic nerve
   e. Common peroneal nerve

5. A 48-year-old male presents with acute pain to his left knee. On examination the knee is swollen, tender and erythematous. You aspirate the knee and results show a white blood cell count of 20,000/mm³ (70% polymorphonuclear neutrophils) and needle-shaped crystals that are negatively birefringent. What type of crystals would likely be present?
   a. Calcium pyrophosphate
   b. Uric acid
   c. Monosodium urate
   d. Calcium phosphate
   e. Cholesterol

6. After a difficult labour, an 8-month-old child presents with an adducted and internally rotated arm with the forearm pronated. A diagnosis of Erb's palsy is made. From which part of the brachial plexus does the nerves of this injury arise from?
   a. Middle trunk
   b. Superior trunk

    c. Inferior trunk
    d. Posterior cord
    e. Medial cord

7. A 17-year-old male falls on to his outstretched hand. On examination there is tenderness in the anatomical snuffbox. Which of the following forms the medial border of the snuffbox?
    a. Abductor pollicis longus
    b. Extensor pollicis brevis
    c. Scaphoid
    d. Extensor pollicis longus
    e. Trapezium

EMQ

For each of the following questions, select the most appropriate answer.

Each option may be used once, more than once or not at all.

  A. Musculocutaneous nerve
  B. Median nerve
  C. Suprascapular nerve
  D. Ulnar nerve
  E. Axillary nerve
  F. Posterior interosseous nerve
  G. Long thoracic nerve
  H. Deep branch of ulnar nerve
  I. Radial nerve
  J. Lower subscapular nerve

8. A 28-year-old female presents with proximal forearm pain. On examination the patient is unable to extend the thumb and other digits at the metacarpophalangeal joints. There is also weak abduction of the thumb. Which nerve is likely affected?

9. A 60-year-old female presents with weakness in her hands. On examination she is unable to adduct and abduct her fingers. You perform a Froment's test and it is positive. Which nerve is likely affected?

10. A 23-year-old athlete presents with pain around his scapula. On examination there is wasting below the spine of the scapula with weak external rotation. Which nerve is likely affected?

Chapter 12

REPRODUCTIVE SYSTEM

1. A 52-year-old male presents in your clinic enquiring about a vasectomy.
   a. Label on the following histology a Leydig cell and seminiferous tubules (2)

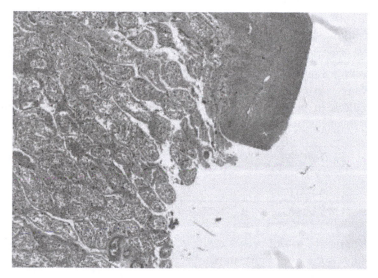

   b. What hormones bind to Leydig and Sertoli cells? (2)
   c. What is the eventual consequence of hormone binding to Leydig and Sertoli cells? (2)
   d. Describe the course of the vas deferens (2)
   e. When performing a vasectomy, what layers do you cut through? (2)

2. A 67-year-old female presents to you complaining of a lump in her right breast. She has noticed no discharge and does not complain of any pain or swelling around the area.
   a. Name two common causes for a lump in the breast in:
      i. An under 20-year-old (1)
      ii. An over 65-year-old (1)
   b. What is the lymphatic drainage of the breasts? (2)
   c. What histological changes would be seen in the breast tissue during pregnancy due to oestrogen and progesterone? (2)
   d. Why do breasts not secrete milk until after birth? (1)
   e. Why is a woman who has had no children and a long gap between menarche and menopause at risk of breast cancer? (1)
   f. The patient went for breast screening which was sensitive and specific. Define sensitivity and specificity (2)

3. A 30-year-old woman who is approximately 26 weeks of gestation presents to you for a review. She is known to drink alcohol every day.
   a. State four investigations/assessments that are performed at any antenatal clinic and indicate what is measured (4)
   b. What effects would drinking have on pregnancy and how does this occur? (2)
   c. What is pre-eclampsia? (1)
   d. State two features or clinical signs that can be seen with pre-eclampsia? (1)
   e. Give two disadvantages of health education to patients regarding drinking during pregnancy (2)

4. A 25-year-old female presents to you complaining of not having had a period for 4 months.
   a. Name two other common causes of secondary amenorrhoea for her age (2)
   b. Indicate in the table below whether the level of oestrogen and progesterone in the menstrual cycle at Day 7, 14 and 21 is low, rising or high (3)

Day	Oestrogen	Progesterone
7		
14		
21		

   c. What is the role of progesterone in early pregnancy for metabolism? (1)
   d. What is the role of human placental lactogen in pregnancy for metabolism? (2)
   e. The patient is found to be pregnant. She undergoes prenatal screening for Down's syndrome with the quadruple test. Name two markers included in this test (2)

5. A 20-week-gestation patient attends the antenatal clinic and undergoes an ultrasound assessment.
   a. In this assessment, what measurement is used to determine the gestational age of foetus in:
      i. First trimester (1)
      ii. Second trimester (1)
   b. Which palpable structure is used to measure symphysis-fundal height? (1)
   c. Explain how amniotic fluid is produced and resorbed in the third trimester (2)
   d. What is the clinical term for excessive amniotic fluid? (1)

   The baby is born and experiences projectile vomiting upon feeding. He fails to pass meconium. Duodenal atresia is diagnosed.

   e. Name two other places that atresia can occur in the gastrointestinal tract, and what may have caused the defect embryologically (2)
   f. Name two other causes for excessive amniotic fluid other than duodenal atresia (2)

6. A 60-year-old female presents to you complaining of postmenopausal bleeding. She has a history of irregular menstrual cycles and has a BMI of 33.
   a. What changes occur in the ovary that induce menopause? (2)
   b. Which layer is involved in menstruation? Label this on the diagram (2)

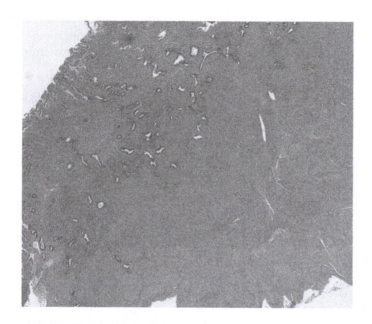

   c. Name two effects of oestrogen on this tissue (2)
   d. How does her BMI contribute to increased risk of endometrial carcinoma? (2)
   e. Explain the rationale for an abdominal hysterectomy with bilateral salpingo-oophorectomy for this patient (2)

7. A 22-year-old female presents to you with right upper quadrant pain. She has sexual intercourse frequently but does not always use barrier contraception. You suspect she has pelvic inflammatory disease (PID).
   a. State and explain a likely cause for the right upper quadrant pain considering the information above (2)
   b. Name the two groups of peritoneal recesses. Why are they clinically significant? (2)
   c. Other than pelvic pain, name two symptoms associated with PID (1)
   d. Name two common organisms that can cause PID (1)
   e. In suspected PID, what routine tests may be recommended in routine clinical practice to confirm diagnosis? (1)
   f. State another routine bedside test that should be done (1)
   g. Name two complications of unresolved PID (2)

8. A 19-week-gestation patient presents to your clinic concerned about foetal development.
   a. Name three factors that are measured on a biophysical profile (3)
   b. Explain with reference to the stages of the respiratory system development why a foetus is not viable at 18 weeks but is at 28 weeks (3)
   c. What is asymmetrical growth restriction and the common cause? (2)
   d. What are the precise actions of oxytocin on the myometrium? (1)
   e. What two landmarks are used to work out the anteroposterior diameter of the pelvic inlet? (1)

9. A young couple presents to your clinic concerned about infertility. They explain they have been trying to conceive for the past year without any success despite having regular sexual intercourse.
   a. What proportion of couples having regular unprotected sexual intercourse would normally be expected to conceive within a year? (1)
   b. Anovulation is a cause of infertility. Name two anovulatory causes (1)
   c. You investigate both partners and ask for a semen sample. What sperm count would you regard as too low for reliable fertility, and what is the normal volume of ejaculate? (2)
   d. Suggest two other characteristics of sperm that are relevant to fertility (2)
   e. Within a few months, she becomes pregnant. The test for human pregnancy is based upon detection of what hormone in the urine? (1)
   f. What structure produces the above hormone in the initial stages of pregnancy? To which stage of pregnancy does the highest level of this hormone correlate and what is its function? (3)

10. A 30-year-old female who is six weeks pregnant presented to A&E with vaginal spotting about an hour ago. She complains of sharp abdominal pain that radiates to the shoulder. You suspect she has an ectopic pregnancy.
    a. Briefly describe the three stages of implantation (3)
    b. State a common site where ectopic pregnancy occurs (1)
    c. Name two predisposing factors that increase the risk of ectopic pregnancy (1)

    The patient later presents with dizziness and profuse sweating. Her blood pressure is 95/60 mmHg, heart rate is 110 bpm, pulse is weak, she has cold peripheries and she is bleeding profusely.

    d. What do you think has happened now? Why can ectopic pregnancy lead to these clinical features? (1)
    e. Explain the mechanism behind why severe blood loss would cause the patient to have cold hands, a fast heart rate and sweating (4)

MCQ

For the following questions, select the single best answer.

1. Which embryonic structure is the female uterus and vagina developed from?
   a. Paramesonephric duct
   b. Wolffian duct
   c. Urogenital sinus
   d. Pronephric duct
   e. Notochord

2. A 17-year-old girl presents with 3-day history of yellow vaginal discharge. She also complains of dysuria and has recently come back from holiday where she had unprotected sex. You decide to treat the patient for gonorrhoea. Which other infection would you treat for while waiting for microbiology results?
   a. Syphilis
   b. Herpes simplex virus
   c. Herpes papillomavirus
   d. Chlamydia
   e. HIV

3. A 35-year-old female presents to A&E following a road traffic accident. She has sustained an unstable pelvis fracture and requires surgery. Which of the following structure DOES NOT pass through the greater sciatic foramen?
   a. Piriformis
   b. Pudendal nerve
   c. Posterior femoral cutaneous nerve
   d. Tendon of obturator internus
   e. Nerve to quadratus femoris

4. A 52-year-old obese female presents complaining of postmenopausal bleeding. She has been taking oestrogen-only hormone replacement therapy for the past 30 years. What is the histology of the cancer she is at risk of?
   a. Squamous cell carcinoma
   b. Transitional cell carcinoma
   c. Basal cell carcinoma
   d. Sarcoma
   e. Adenocarcinoma

5. You are teaching the physiology of the male reproductive system. Which of the following is the correct pathway for sperm release?
   a. Testes → vas deferens → epididymis → prostate gland → seminal vesicle → urethra
   b. Testes →epididymis → vas deferens → prostate gland → seminal vesicle → urethra

   c. Testes → epididymis → prostate gland → vas deferens →
      seminal vesicle → urethra
   d. Testes → seminal vesicle → epididymis → vas deferens →
      prostate gland → urethra
   e. Testes → seminal vesicle → vas deferens → epididymis →
      prostate gland → urethra

6. A 28-year-old girl presents with dyspareunia. She also complains that she
   has seen a lump near the vaginal opening which is painful. On examination
   you notice a fluid-like swelling on her labia majora. Which is the lymphatic
   drainage of this anatomical structure?
   a. Internal iliac os
   b. External iliac nodes
   c. Obturator nodes
   d. Superficial femoral nodes
   e. Superficial inguinal nodes

7. A couple visits the clinic concerned about infertility. You undertake
   investigations for both the husband and wife and results from the husband's
   semen analysis shows an abnormality. Which of the following is NOT a
   parameter within normal range?
   a. Volume 2.5 ml
   b. Total motility 50%
   c. Sperm concentration 10,000,000/ml
   d. Progressive motility 45%
   e. Vitality 70% live

EMQ

For each of the following questions, select the most appropriate answer.

Each option may be used once, more than once or not at all.

  A. Day 10
  B. Day 13
  C. Day 15
  D. Inhibin
  E. Luteinising hormone
  F. Follicle-stimulating hormone
  G. Oestrogen
  H. Progesterone
  I. Prolactin
  J. Human chorionic gonadotropin

8. The decrease of which hormone level is responsible for the contraction of
   spiral arteries in the functional endometrium?

9. Luteinising hormone surge occurs on which day?

10. Theca interna cells express receptors for which hormone?

Chapter 13

NERVOUS SYSTEM

1. A 55-year-old male presents to A&E with weakness in his right arm and leg. There is also reduced tactile sensation on his right arm and leg.
   a. Which brain side is affected and why? (2)
   b. Name the two most common causes (2)
   c. How and where is cerebrospinal fluid produced and reabsorbed? (2)
   d. You undertake a neurological exam on this patient. State the nerve roots tested for each reflex.
      i. Biceps (1)
      ii. Ankle jerk (1)
      iii. Patellar reflex (1)
   e. Describe what you would expect the muscle tone to be in the right and left arms (1)

2. A 39-year-old male presents to you with unsteady gait and balance. He has been drinking alcohol heavily since the age of 13.
   a. What is the most likely explanation for this man's presentation? (1)
   b. Describe how alcohol is metabolised (2)
   c. Label the following structure of the brain (3)

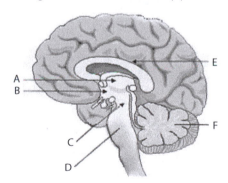

   d. Name the classic triad of signs of cerebellar disease (1)
   e. Neurones within the central nervous system do not regenerate whereas peripheral nervous system (PNS) regeneration is possible following neuronal damage. Outline the mechanisms for neuronal repair in PNS (3)

3. A wife of a 63-year-old male has noticed he has an expressionless face, shaking of his hands and difficulty moving. A diagnosis of Parkinson's disease is made.
   a. Describe the diagnostic characteristics/classical signs you would expect to see as the patient walks towards a chair (2)
   b. Give two other signs which would support the diagnosis of Parkinson's disease (2)

    c. Which part of the brain is most likely affected in Parkinson's disease? Describe its anatomy and state two functions (4)

    d. Give two treatments for Parkinson's disease and briefly describe its mechanism of action (2)

4. A 28-year-old female presents to A&E following a motorcycle accident which has resulted in head trauma.

    a. A CT scan reveals an expanding brain haematoma. Name two possible ocular signs that the patient may present with (2)

    b. Name and describe two anatomical haemorrhages in the skull (4)

    c. A bloodstained watery fluid is leaking from her ear. What is this called? (1)

    d. Which bone has fractured? (1)

    e. Which two cranial nerves should be tested? (2)

5. You review a patient in A&E who you suspect has a spinal cord lesion.

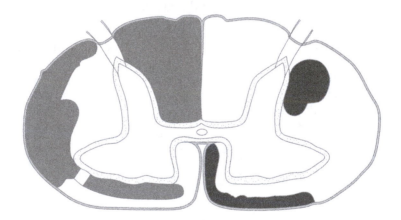

    a. Identify on the diagram above where you would find tracts for pain, temperature and crude touch perception and label them (2)

    b. On which side of the body would these tracts correspond to? (1)

    c. Identify on the diagram where you find lateral corticospinal tracts. Label this and state to which side this corresponds (2)

    d. You elicit that this patient has spastic paraparesis of the right side, with brisk reflexes and up going plantar reflex. On the left side there is loss of temperature sensation and no plantar reflex. Which side of the spinal cord is the lesion? (1)

    e. Why is there no plantar reflex on the left side? (1)

    f. What type of motor neurone lesion does the above suggest? (1)

    g. What type of motor neurone lesion would cause fasciculations? Suggest another neurological finding (1)

    h. Why would it be better to arrange for an MRI rather than a CT scan in this case? (1)

6. A man presents to hospital having fainted earlier today. He had experienced slurred speech shortly after but seems to have fully recovered and insists he is fine.
   a. What is the most likely cause of this man's symptoms? (1)
   b. Why is secondary prevention important in this patient? (1)
   c. What class of pharmaceutical agent should be used for secondary prevention? (1)
   d. State what is the most likely imaging technique likely to be carried out for this patient (1)
   e. During his symptoms, he seemed to understand what was being said, but found it difficult to express himself. What type of aphasia is this? (1)
   f. Where in the anatomy of the cortex is this area? (1)
   g. What is the blood supply to this area? (1)
   h. Explain why this man only experienced the symptoms for a short while but now seems fully recovered (1)
   i. What two pieces of advice would you give to this patient with a group one driving licence? (2)

7. An 80-year-old man comes to see you in the memory clinic. A diagnosis of frontotemporal dementia is made.
   a. Give four personality/behavioural changes in this patient due to frontal lobe atrophy (2)
   b. The patient later presents with tremors, rigidity and myoclonic jerks. Explain why (1)
   c. State the pathology that could affect the blood vessel that supplies the frontal lobe (1)
   d. Normal pressure hydrocephalus (NPH) is another cause of dementia. Briefly explain what this is (2)
   e. What is the classic triad related to this condition? (3)
   f. How can NPH be surgically managed? (1)

8. A 70-year-old male has a slip and fall at home. His CT head scan is below:

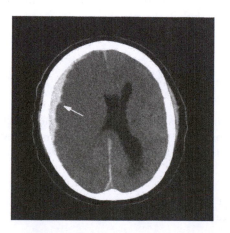

a. Describe the image above (1)
b. Between which two layers is a subdural haematoma formed? (1)
c. Which type of vessels may be involved in this type of haemorrhage, and which local circulation does it contribute to? (2)
d. The patient initially collapses at home. He was later brought to the hospital and regains consciousness. The GCS was 15/15. A few hours later, he started to deteriorate and the GCS started to drop. What is the preferred clinical neurological term used to describe the short period of full consciousness? (1)
e. Give two reasons why this type of haemorrhage tends to occur in the elderly (2)
f. Give one suggestion of treatment to save this patient's life (1)
g. Coning/tonsillar herniation may be a potential complication of the above. Describe what this is (2)

MCQ

For the following questions, select the single best answer.

1. You are conducting an experiment between two drugs for the treatment of multiple sclerosis. Drug A has shown to increase the length constant of the axon compared to drug B. What effect would this have on the action potential travelling down the axon?
   a. No change
   b. Slower
   c. Faster
   d. Smaller diameter
   e. None of the above

2. A 35-year-old intravenous drug user has a diagnosis of infective endocarditis. He develops neurological deficits specifically with spatial recognition. There is a suspicion of a central nervous system (CNS) complication and a brain MRI scan reveals an abscess. Which part of the brain is most frequently affected by septic emboli in this patient?
   a. Parietal lobe
   b. Frontal lobe
   c. Occipital lobe
   d. Temporal lobe
   e. Cerebellum

3. A 28-year-old female presents with a seizure. She describes of having thoughts where ordinary objects and words seem somewhat different than they would normally feel but not unfamiliar. What type of experience is she describing?
   a. Jamais vu
   b. Hallucination
   c. Retrograde amnesia

d. Delusion

e. Déjà vu

4. A 40-year-old male presents with recurrent ulcers over the feet over the past 9 months. He now complains of ataxia, inability to see distant objects, tingling and numbness and weakness in the lower limbs. On examination temperature, pain and fine touch sensations were normal but crude touch sensations was decreased below the T12 level. Vibration sense, tactile localisation, tactile discrimination and joint position sense were lost on both sides below the knees. Which organism is responsible for this presentation?

a. Mycobacterium tuberculosis

b. Borrelia burgdorferi

c. Cryptococcal meningitis

d. Taenia solium

e. Treponema pallidum

5. A 35-year-old female with a background of multiple sclerosis presents with unilateral optic neuritis and rapid decrease in central vision. Where does a central scotoma suggest a lesion is located?

a. Optic nerve

b. Optic chiasm

c. Optic tract

d. Macula

e. Temporal lobe lesion

6. A 30-year-old male is diagnosed with syringomyelia. An MRI scan shows a syrinx pressing on the ventral white commissure. On examination which function deficit would you expect to see?

a. Ipsilateral loss of temperature and pain sensations

b. Contralateral loss of temperature and pain sensations

c. Ipsilateral loss of tactile sensation and proprioception

d. Ipsilateral loss of muscle co-ordination

e. None of the above

7. A 45-year-old female presents with a decreased level of consciousness, dysphagia, dysarthria and contralateral limb weakness. You suspect a brain stem injury and undertake a cranial nerve examination. You brush the cornea lightly with a fine wisp of cotton and there is an absence of blinking. Which cranial nerves are tested in this reflex?

a. Cranial nerves III + IV

b. Cranial nerves V + VII

c. Cranial nerves IV and VI

d. Cranial nerves IX and X

e. Cranial nerves VII and IX

EMQ

For each of the following questions, select the most appropriate answer.

Each option may be used once, more than once or not at all.

A. Lateral horn of the spinal cord
B. Dorsal root ganglia
C. Anterior horn of spinal cord
D. Corticospinal tracts
E. Posterior column tract
F. Spinocerebellar tract
G. Vestibulospinal tract
H. Medulla
I. Brainstem
J. Spinal cord

8. A patient presents with weakness, fasciculations and atrophy of the limb muscles, without any sensory loss. Where is the likely damage?

9. At what level does the dorsal column medial lemniscus decussate?

10. With regard to the spinothalamic tract, where does the first order neuron travel through and synapse?

Chapter 14

HEAD AND NECK

1. A man with left-sided weakness presents with an inability to blink his left eye, left mouth drooping and left cheek paralysis. His GP suspects facial nerve lesion.
   a. Why can't he blink? (1)
   b. Which muscle opens the eye and will that be affected? Why? (2)
   c. What quick test or examination could be done in the GP practice to help determine whether this man has an upper or lower motor neurone lesion? (1)
   d. Why does he still have taste in the anterior two-thirds of his tongue? (1)
   e. What is the sensation pattern to the anterior two-third and posterior third of the tongue? (1)
   f. Name the pharyngeal arch that the facial nerve is associated with (1)
   g. Give three muscle structures that are derived from this pharyngeal arch (3)

2. A boy is hit in the face and sustains a fracture of medial and inferior walls of the orbit.
   a. What bones make up medial and lateral walls? (2)
   b. There is an area of paraesthesia over the cheek, lateral sides of the nose and upper lip. Which nerve and branch is affected? (2)
   c. There is blood in the anterior chamber of the eye. What is the medical name for this? (1)
   d. Bulging of the eye is noted. What is the medical name for this? (1)
   e. Which structure produces aqueous humour and what is the drainage pathway? (3)
   f. Clear fluid leakage is noted from the nose. What substance could this be? (1)

3. A patient presents to your clinic complaining of a lump on his neck. On examination you notice an enlarged lymph node near the external jugular vein
   a. Define dysphagia (1)
   b. Where does the external jugular vein drain? (1)
   c. Why does the thyroid move on swallowing? (2)
   d. What is the arterial supply of the thyroid? (2)
   e. What is the retropharyngeal space? (1) What complications can arise from the spread of infection here? (1)
   f. Give two general reasons or benefits of cervical fascia (2)

4. A 13-month-old boy presents to your clinic with otalgia and pain behind the ear. You notice swelling and tenderness behind his ear.
   a. What do you think this swelling is? (1)
   b. State in general terms the two main components of the inner ear (1)
   c. Through what does the inner ear communicate with the subarachnoid space? (1)
   d. How can middle ear infection spread to the subarachnoid space? (1)
   e. What are the ossicles of the middle ear? (1)
   f. Through what kind of joint do they articulate and what is their function? (2)
   g. Name one muscle of the middle ear that dampens down noise inflicted on the tympanic membrane (1)
   h. Which bones of the ear are derived from the first pharyngeal arch? (2)

5. A 50-year-old woman presents to your clinic with a 3-month history of increasing swelling in the front of her neck. She has noticed that she has been losing weight and is always feeling hot.
   a. Which two cranial nerves innervate the muscles of the pharynx? (2)
   b. Where does the thyroid descend from? (1)
   c. Which two muscles are anterior to the thyroid gland? (2)
   d. What are the potential consequences of calcium and phosphate during thyroid surgery? (2)
   e. Name the cells that secrete parathyroid hormone (1)
   f. During thyroid surgery what nerve could be compressed and what general consequence would that produce? (2)

6. A 2-year-old child presents to your clinic feeling generally unwell – earache, fever and hearing loss.
   a. Name three aggregates of lymphoid tissue in the pharynx (3)
   b. Which one of these will cause infection to the ear? (1)
   c. In which part of the cranium do you find the middle ear? (1)
   d. Name two reasons that a middle ear infection can cause loss of hearing (2)
   e. What two spaces communicate with the middle ear? (2)
   f. Why are children more likely to get middle ear infections when they have upper respiratory tract infection? (1)

7. A 22-year-old female presents with extreme jaw pain which projects to her ears. This pain is worse when she moves her jaw and she is able to hear clicking and popping.
   a. What type of joint is the temporomandibular joint? (1)
   b. Name the three ligaments associated with the temporomandibular joint (3)
   c. The temporomandibular joint capsule is divided into superior and inferior compartments. What are their actions? (2)
   d. Which muscles elevate the mandible and what nerve supplies them? (2)
   e. The nerve mentioned in answer (d) is associated with which embryonic derivative? (be precise) (1)
   f. Inflammation at the temporomandibular joint and associated nerve entrapment causes loss of innervations to which part of the tongue? (1)

8. A 90-year-old male with a background of cardiovascular disease has sudden painless unilateral loss of vision. On examination his visual acuity is markedly reduced to only counting fingers.
   a. What is the arterial supply to the eye? (1)
   b. What is the likely diagnosis? Briefly explain the pathophysiology (3)
   c. What structure does the artery and vein run through to supply the inner layer of the eye? (1)
   d. Name two orbital causes of papilloedema (2)
   e. With regard to his age what are the two most common causes of reduced vision? (2)
   f. Why would a cranial nerve three palsy cause ptosis? (1)

9. A 50-year-old male with a 30 pack-year history presents with a lump in the left supraclavicular region, hoarseness and a weak cough. Over the years he has mainly produced clear sputum. Examination reveals a fixed irregular mass behind the medial end of the left clavicle, left ptosis and unequal pupils.
   a. Explain the ptosis (1)
   b. Explain the unequal pupils. Which pupil would you expect to be larger? (2)
   c. What would be the finding on testing the light reflex? (2)
   d. Explain the likely findings on examination of the larynx. (2)
   e. Explain the reason for the weak cough (2)
   f. What is the most likely type of lung cancer histologically giving a pancoast tumour? (1)

10. A 6-year-old boy presents a constant runny nose. The parents have noticed that he is snoring at night and there is noisy breathing through the nose. On examination you notice he has enlarged adenoids.
    a. Where are the adenoids located? (1)
    b. Which type of epithelium are the adenoids lined with? (1)
    c. Which surrounding structure may be obstructed? (1)
    d. Give three specific consequence of this condition (3)
    e. The doctor recognised it as a viral infection. Give one common viral agent which could cause this (1)
    f. Name a bacterial agent that may cause adenoiditis, and comment on its gram staining (1)
    g. The patient undergoes an adenoidectomy. Name two potential complications (2)

MCQ

For the following questions, select the single best answer.

1. A patient is diagnosed with a staphylococcus infection of the frontal sinuses. By which route is this infection likely to reach the brain?
   a. Subclavian artery
   b. Cavernous sinus

   c. Vertebral artery

   d. Inferior sagittal sinus

   e. Superior sagittal sinus

2. A 40-year-old female presents with a swollen neck. On examination there is a firm thyroid mass, which moved upward with swallowing. This occurs due to the thyroid gland being invested by which fascia?
   a. Superficial cervical facia
   b. Investing layer of deep cervical fascia
   c. Prevertebral fascia
   d. Carotid sheath
   e. Pretracheal fascia

3. Which of the following nerve innervates the muscles of mastication?
   a. Mandibular nerve
   b. Ophthalmic nerve
   c. Maxillary nerve
   d. Facial nerve
   e. Vagus nerve

4. A 55-year-old male complains of electrical shock attacks upon swallowing. He describes the pain being felt in the back of the throat and tongue. Which nerve is responsible for the innervation of the pain he experiences?
   a. Hypoglossal nerve
   b. Chorda tympani
   c. Glossopharyngeal nerve
   d. Lingual nerve
   e. Internal laryngeal nerve

5. A 28-year-old male suffers a trauma injury and presents with ptosis of the lid, exophthalmos, ophthalmoplegia, fixation and dilatation of the pupil and loss of sensitivity to the upper eyelid and forehead. There is no deficit in visual acuity. Which of the following is the likely cause for this presentation?
   a. Cavernous artery aneurysm
   b. Sarcoidosis
   c. Giant cell arteritis
   d. Superior orbital fissure syndrome
   e. Orbital apex syndrome

6. A 38-year-old female presents complaining of dry eyes and reduced nasal and lacrimal gland secretions. Where is the lesion most likely located?
   a. Ciliary ganglion
   b. Pterygopalatine ganglion
   c. Submandibular ganglion
   d. Otic ganglion
   e. None of the above

7. A 22-year-old singer complains of losing her higher vocal registers. A diagnosis of superior laryngeal nerve injury is confirmed. Which of the following muscles does this nerve innervate?
   a. Cricothyroid
   b. Posterior cricoarytenoid
   c. Lateral cricoarytenoid
   d. Arytenoid
   e. Aryepiglottic

EMQ

For each of the following questions, select the most appropriate answer.

Each option may be used once, more than once or not at all.

A. Supraorbital foramen
B. Foramen caecum
C. Superior orbital fissure
D. Stylomastoid foramen
E. Foramen sphenopalatinum
F. Foramen ovale
G. Foramen spinosum
H. Foramen lacerum
I. Jugular foramen
J. Foramen magnum

8. A patient presents with hoarseness of voice, deviation of uvula towards the normal side, loss of taste from posterior third of the tongue and sternocleidomastoid, and trapezius muscle paresis. The lesion is likely to be obstructing which foramen?

9. A patient suffers a traumatic head injury and a CT scan shows an epidural haematoma. Which foramen contains the origin of the vessel that contributes to the majority of these bleeds?

10. A patient presents with right-sided facial drooping and drooping of the eyelid. You suspect he has Bell's palsy. The nerve that is affected in this condition leaves the skull at which foramen?

Chapter 15

CLINICAL PHARMACOLOGY

1. A 55-year-old female with rheumatoid arthritis presents to your clinic with worsening symptoms. She has already tried a combination of methotrexate and sulfasalazine. You decide to initiate her on ciclosporin.
   a. What is the mechanism of action of ciclosporin? (2)
   b. Name two factors affecting oral bioavailability (2)
   c. NSAIDs may be used to help manage pain and inflammation. Name the enzyme inhibited for therapeutic effect. Which is responsible for adverse drug reactions? (2)
   d. Pharmacodynamically, how does an NSAID cause its therapeutic effects? (2)
   e. Name two G-protein receptor subtypes which are acted upon by prostaglandins to cause increased pain or pyrexia (2)

2. A 35-year-old male patient presents to your clinic complaining of lower back pain. He has already tried paracetamol and ibuprofen with no effect. You decide to prescribe him codeine.
   a. Describe the mechanism of codeine in terms of its pharmacokinetics (2)
   b. Opiates act on receptors which are G-protein coupled. Name the three main types (3)
   c. What effects do opiates have on the postsynaptic membrane? (1)
   d. Define ED_{50} and LD_{50} (2)
   e. Apart from death, name another important adverse effect with opiate overdose? (1)
   f. How would you treat opiate overdose? (1)

3. A 40-year-old female presents to A&E with paracetamol overdose. She states she has taken a single dose of 40 tablets with a bottle of wine seven hours ago.
   a. How is paracetamol metabolised in a normal patient? (2)
   b. How would it be metabolised differently in an overdosed patient? (1)
   c. Would this patient require treatment? Explain your answer (3)
   d. What is first-line treatment for paracetamol overdose, and how would you administer it? (2)
   e. Sketch a graph for a drug that shows first-order kinetics in elimination (2)

4. A 32-year-old female is admitted into the psychiatry unit for assessment. You determine that she has persistent hallucinations with thought disorder and suspect she has schizophrenia. You initiate her on olanzapine.
   a. What is the mechanism of action of this drug? (2)
   b. The side effects of drugs to treat schizophrenia may mimic what condition? (1)

   c. Name two other side effects of this drug (2)

   d. Some symptoms of schizophrenia can be due to a defect in the serotonin pathway. Name two behavioural symptoms/signs of schizophrenia (2)

   e. Fluoxetine is given to treat the above. Name the class and action of this drug (2)

   f. Why might it be particularly important to monitor young adult patients at the beginning of treatment with a selective serotonin reuptake inhibitor, or if a dosage is changed? (1)

5. A 23-year-old female diagnosed with epilepsy since childhood comes to your clinic. She is on carbamazepine but has been having seizures as of late. She is a heavy drinker.

   a. Give two potential precipitants to seizures in this patient (2)

   b. What types of epilepsy are treated with carbamazepine? (1)

   c. What main class of drugs does this belong to? (1)

   d. What is the mechanism of action of carbamazepine? (2)

   e. What needs to be considered in this patient when taking this drug in terms of interactions with other drugs and half-life? (2)

   f. The patient states she wishes to have a baby. Which antiepileptic should be avoided and why? (2)

6. A 25-year-old male presents with bloody diarrhoea for the past month with weight loss and fever. He is diagnosed with inflammatory bowel disease.

   a. State one endoscopic feature each for ulcerative colitis and Crohn's disease (2)

   b. The patient is tested for perinuclear anti-neutrophil cytoplasmic antibodies (pANCA). In which inflammatory disease would it be positive? (1)

   c. The patient develops red rounded nodules on his shins. What is this? (1)

   d. Name another skin problem associated with inflammatory bowel disease (1)

   e. Patient is diagnosed with ulcerative colitis and given medication but develops recurrent urinary tract infections. Why is this? (1)

   f. Name a drug to control fever (1). Briefly describe its mechanism of action (1)

   g. Name a drug to control fever; briefly describe its mechanism of action (2)

7. A 40-year-old male presents with burning retrosternal discomfort after meals and constant belching.

   a. What is the mechanism of a protein pump inhibitor? (2)

   b. This does not seem to be working. Name an alternative drug you could try and its mechanism of action (2)

   c. Name two gastrointestinal side effects associated with protein pump inhibitors (2)

   d. The yellow card scheme collects information on suspected problems or incidents. Name four elements which are involved (4)

8. A 70-year-old male presents with enlarged, painless non-tender cervical lymph nodes. He also complains of fever and night sweats. Tissue diagnosis has revealed a diagnosis of Hodgkin's lymphoma.

a. On the diagram below indicate the class of cytotoxic agent that would act at each cellular level (4)

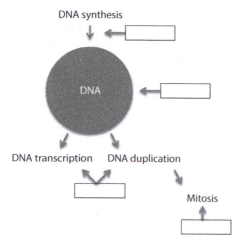

b. Give two patient factors that should be considered before commencing chemotherapy (2)

c. Vincristine is given to the patient. Give the mechanism of this drug (2)

The patient has entered into a trial of a new chemotherapy drug, which is given once a day with a half-life of 24 hours.

d. Using this information draw a simple smoothed line plot on the graph below of how plasma levels of this drug would reach steady state (1)

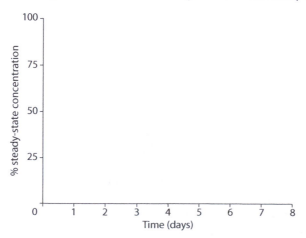

e. Side effects of this drug are experienced when the steady state reaches 75%. On which day would you expect to see these side effects occur? (1)

MCQ

For the following questions, select the single best answer.

1. A 43-year-old female presents with continuous right upper quadrant pain, vomiting and fever. This pain is worse after eating greasy or fatty foods. On examination, Murphy's sign is positive and blood results show an elevated white cell count and a mildly elevated bilirubin. Ultrasound reveals a thick-walled, shrunken gallbladder and a dilated common bile duct. Which of the following analgesia is treatment of choice in this patient?
   a. Morphine
   b. Paracetamol
   c. Pethidine
   d. Oxycodone
   e. Ibuprofen

2. A 52-year-old male with a diagnosis of lymphoma is started on a chemotherapy regimen. Post-treatment he complains of gross haematuria and dysuria. Which of the following drugs is responsible for this side effect?
   a. Doxorubicin
   b. Vincristine
   c. Prednisone
   d. Cyclophosphamide
   e. Rituximab

3. A 70-year-old male presents with shortness of breath, pitting oedema and pulmonary crackles at the lung bases. A diagnosis of heart failure is confirmed. Blood results show a potassium of 3.0 mmol/L. Which diuretic would be the treatment of choice?
   a. Spironolactone
   b. Furosemide
   c. Bendroflumethiazide
   d. Bumetanide
   e. Indapamide

4. A 22-year-old female presents with increased urinary frequency, dysuria and urgency. There is no history of recent sexual activity. On examination there is no vaginal discharge, abdominal tenderness or cervical excitation. Dipstick analysis of urine is positive for nitrite and leukocytes. Which of the following initial treatment is most appropriate?
   a. Azithromycin
   b. Doxycycline
   c. Fluconazole
   d. Cefotaxime
   e. Trimethoprim

5. A 32-year-old female presents to A&E with diplopia, bradycardia, hypotension and increased respiratory rate. She has a background of mental health problems and has taken an overdose of diazepam with alcohol. Which immediate medication would you administer to her?
   a. Naloxone
   b. Flumazenil
   c. Protamine
   d. Deferoxamine

6. A 68-year-old male presents to your clinic for an INR check following a stroke 2 weeks ago. He has a background of heartburn and peptic ulcers. His INR reading shows 4.2. Which of the following medications is responsible for this high INR reading?
   a. Omeprazole
   b. Lansoprazole
   c. Cimetidine
   d. Gaviscon
   e. Ranitidine

7. A new hypertensive medication has shown promising results in clinical trials. The pharmacokinetic profile shows a half-life of 8 hours. If this drug was given as a continuous infusion, how long would it take to reach 75% of steady state?
   a. 8 hours
   b. 16 hours
   c. 4 hours
   d. 24 hours
   e. 32 hours

EMQ

For each of the following questions, select the most appropriate answer.

Each option may be used once, more than once or not at all.

A. Amoxicillin
B. Erythromycin
C. Cephalexin
D. Ciprofloxacin
E. Rifampicin
F. Trimethoprim
G. Gentamicin
H. Linezolid
I. Tigecycline
J. Clotrimazole

8. Which antibiotic works by binding irreversibly to a site on the 50S subunit of the bacterial ribosome thereby inhibiting protein synthesis?

9. An 18-year-old female has a positive pregnancy test. She is surprised as she has been taking the combined oral contraceptive but mentions that she has been on a 2-week course of antibiotics. Which antibiotic is likely to have caused this?

10. A patient is started on an antibiotic for the treatment of sepsis. He later complains of hearing loss with vertigo. Which antibiotic is responsible for this side effect?

Chapter 16

SOCIETY AND MEDICINE

1. A local paper has recently decided to take an interest in multiple sclerosis (MS) and sends a reporter over to interview you. The reporter asks you about the incidence and prevalence of the condition.
   a. Define the terms incidence and prevalence (2)
   b. From June 2013 to November 2014, 600 new cases of MS in a population of 500,000 were reported. Calculate the incidence rate (2)
   c. If the reporter asks you what effect a cure would have on the incidence and prevalence of MS, what would you say? (1)
   d. The prevalence of MS increased greatly over the last century, though its incidence did not. Give the single reason why this most probably occurred. Suggest another reason how prevalence can increase (2)
   e. A later study reports that the probability of being alive 10 years after diagnosis of MS is higher on a new treatment than on conventional therapy. The paper reports an odds ratio of 1.5 (95% CI 0.5–2.5). Explain what this means and explain the implications for the new treatment (2)
   f. Explain the term intention to treat (1)

2. The number of patients diagnosed with bladder cancer, who regularly smoke cigarettes, has increased from 15% in 2000 to 30% in 2003. A journalist questions you and asks what are the intentions of the Department of Health with regard to this 'worrying two-fold increase'.
   a. Do these data provide convincing evidence of a link between cigarette smoking and bladder cancer? Answer yes or no and give the single major argument which supports your answer (2)
   b. The Department of Health decides to investigate matters further and gives you 3 months to carry out a study to investigate the possible link in more detail. You quickly find out that there are no helpful routine data. What sort of study would you carry out? Give two advantages of this design (3)
   c. A study in Canada has shown that among cigarette smokers there are three new cases of bladder cancer in 100,000 person years. Among non-smokers there are 12 new cases in 1,000,000 person years. What is the incidence rate ratio? (1)
   d. The error factor is approximately 3.5. What is the 95% confidence interval? (2)
   e. A representative from a cigarette company is completely reassured, because this result is 'not statistically significant' (p>0.05) Do you agree that this is 'not statistically significant'? Give one reason for your answer (2)

3. A case-control study was conducted to establish the relationship between the use of conjugated oestrogens and the risk of endometrial cancer. Below are the results of the study:

Odds ratio = 2.23, 95% Confidence interval = 1.73–2.73, p = 0.0001

   a. Explain the results from this case-control study (3)
   b. Describe two advantages and two disadvantages of case-control studies compared to cohort studies (4)
   c. What would be the response of somebody if they were told they had cancer? (2)
   d. What is the role of the National Standard Framework? (1)

4. Your consultant suspects your region has a higher prevalence of children with asthma. She wants you to design a survey.
   a. Name two elements to consider when conducting research in children (2)
   b. The incidence rate ratio for children treated in this region is higher than the rest of the country for the general population. Does this mean that your consultant was right in her suspicions? (2)
   c. Parents think that the reason their children have asthma is because of the rape seed oil cultivation nearby. How would know if this is right? (2)

   You come across a recently published large randomised controlled trial which shows a particular ineffective treatment. However, your colleague disagrees with this result as he has decided to follow up on the recommendation from a systematic review.

   d. Do you agree with your colleague's comment? Explain why (4)

5. The incidence of death and admission to hospital due to colon cancer is shown in the table below:

	Unadjusted relative risk (95% confidence interval)	Adjusted relative risk (95% confidence interval)
Meat, fish and vegetables	1.00	1.00
Fish and vegetables	0.86	0.91 (0.73–1.15)
Vegetarian or vegan	0.60	0.69 (0.65–0.86)

Adjusted for sex, smoking, education level, long-term medical treatment
   a. Name one genetic condition that is associated with an increased chance of colon cancer (1)
   b. Explain one study design of a prospective and retrospective cohort study (2)
   c. Comment on the adjusted relative risk of a vegetarian diet (2)

d. The patient's partner is worried about getting colon cancer.
   He is considering taking a fish and vegetable diet. Is there any
   reduction in risk of developing colon cancer if he opts for this diet?
   Explain why (2)
e. Give two reasons why randomised controlled trials are prone to losses
   to follow-up (2)
f. What is a confounding factor? (1)

MCQ

For the following questions, select the single best answer.

1. A new antibody test has been developed for the detection of prostate
   cancer. From the results below, what is the sensitivity of this test?

	Prostate cancer positive	Prostate cancer negative
Antibody test positive	150	95
Antibody test negative	70	350

   a. 61%
   b. 85%
   c. 79%
   d. 68%
   e. 33%

2. A new screening test has been developed for the detection of Crohn's
   disease. A total of 1300 people were tested and results are shown below.
   What is the specificity of this test?

	Positive screening test	Negative screening test	Total
Crohn's disease	200	50	250
No Crohn's disease	350	700	1050
Total	550	750	1300

   a. 200/250
   b. 700/1050
   c. 700/750
   d. 220/550
   e. None of the above

3. A study is conducted on the high-density lipoprotein (HDL) level in the blood
   on a special diet. Only those candidates who have an HDL level at least two
   standard deviations above the mean of 4.5 mmol/L are eligible for the study.
   From a population study of 100, how many are eligible for the study?
   a. 2.5
   b. 5

c. 1.25

d. 10

e. 7.5

4. There has been a recent outbreak of tuberculosis (TB) in the local area. A study has been conducted to find out the prevalence of TB within the local community, which has a population of 200,000 people. A total of 60 people have been identified to have the condition. What is the point prevalence of TB in this population at this given time?

a. 0.3 per 100,000

b. 3 per 100,000

c. 300 per 100,000

d. 0.03 per 100,000

e. 30 per 100,000

5. A study is conducted to determine whether past exposure of cigarette smoking is associated with bladder cancer among people aged 75 and over. Which type of analysis is used in this type of study?

a. Incidence risk ratio

b. Standard mortality ratio

c. Odds ratio

d. Number needed to treat

e. Absolute risk reduction

6. You conduct a study to see the effects of tea on blood pressure. You divide the groups into black tea, green tea and no tea. Which statistical test is most appropriate to test the statistical significance?

a. Student's t-test

b. Chi-square test

c. Fisher's exact test

d. Mann–Whitney U test

e. Analysis of variance (ANOVA)

7. A new treatment has shown to be effective against lung cancer. Clinicians have started to use this new treatment and if all other factors remain unchanged, which of the following is likely to happen?

a. Prevalence will increase

b. Prevalence will decrease

c. Incidence will increase

d. Incidence will decrease

e. Neither prevalence or incidence will be affected

EMQ

For each of the following questions, select the most appropriate answer.

Each option may be used once, more than once or not at all.

A. Case-control study

B. Cohort study

C. Meta-analysis
D. Systematic review
E. Randomised control trial
F. Prevalence survey
G. Paired *t*-test
H. Funnel plot
I. Forest plot
J. Meta-regression

8. You would like to conduct a study to eliminate any confounding factors. Which study design is best suited for this?

9. In terms of time, which study can be conducted either retrospectively or prospectively?

10. Which statistical method is best used to identify publication bias?

Chapter 17

ANSWERS

Cellular Structure and Function (Chapter 1)

1.
   a. Any one of the following scores half a mark: total of one mark.
   Provide support for body structures
   Skin elasticity
   Maintains external and internal structures of cells
   Connects and supports the body organs and various tissues
   b. Collagen is the most abundant protein in the extracellular matrix and hence collagens are the major structural element of all connective tissues and found in the interstitial tissue of virtually all parenchymal organs (1)
   c. Ascorbic acid is required as a cofactor for prolyl hydroxylase and lysyl hydroxylase and these enzymes are responsible for the hydroxylation of the proline and lysine amino acids in collagen. (1) This hydroxylation allows increased H-bonding to stabilise the triple helix. The lack of vitamin C leads to weak tropocollagen triple helices, therefore scurvy (1)
   d. Dominant genetic conditions are conditions that manifest in heterozygotes (individuals with just one mutated copy of the allele) (1)
   e. The assembly of the triple helix requires a glycine residue in every third position along each alpha chain as it is the smallest amino acid. A high content of proline is required to stabilise the structure by allowing hydroxylation (2)
   f. Hydroxylation of proline and lysine residues – intracellularly (1)
   N and C terminal peptides are cleaved and tropocollagen is formed – extracellularly (1)
   Formation of collagen fibrils via covalent cross-linking of adjacent lysine residues – extracellularly (1)

This question is about protein processing and, in particular, collagen. Collagen is the major insoluble fibrous protein in the extracellular matrix and in connective tissue. There are many types of collagen but the majority of the collagen in the body consists of type I, II and III. Collagen-related conditions can arise from genetic or autoimmune defects, nutritional deficiencies which will affect the biosynthesis, assembly, post-translational modification, secretion or other processes involved in collagen production.

This case study describes osteogenesis imperfecta, which is a type 1 collagen defect.

Type I collagen defects cause diseases such as osteogenesis imperfecta. It is a condition that arises due to mutation in the COL1A1 or COL1A2 gene, which encodes the two chains of type 1 collagen. The mutation is due to the substitution of glycine with a bigger amino acid. It is typically characterised by fragile bones that fracture easily, blue sclera, spinal curvature, hearing loss, loose joints and muscle weakness.

Other collagen disorders to be aware of are Ehlers–Danlos syndrome, Alport syndrome and Goodpasture's syndrome.

Insulin is another protein to be aware of in terms of its synthesis and processing.

2.
   a. K_m is the substrate concentration at half the maximum velocity (1)
   b. The active site of an enzyme is the place where substrates bind and where chemical reaction occurs. (1) Active sites have a complementary shape to the substrate therefore upon binding of substrates can induce changes in the conformation and catalysis begins (1)
   c. This is when a molecule binds to an enzyme at a site other than the active site (1)
   d. Phosphofructokinase (PKP) (1) – catalyses the rate-limiting step in glycolysis.
   ATP, citrate or H+ (1) are inhibitors therefore slowing down glycolysis. AMP or fructose-2,6-bisphosphate (Fru-2, 6-P_2) (1) are activators therefore accelerating glycolysis.
   e. PKP catalyses the conversion of fructose-6-phosphate (F6P) and ATP to fructose 1,6-bisphosphate and ADP (1)
   F2, 6BP is a potent activator of PFP and is synthesised when F6P is phosphorylated by phosphofructonase 2. (1) The result of lower levels of liver F2, 6BP is a decrease in activity of PFP and an increase in activity of fructose 1,6-bisphosphate so that gluconeogenesis is favoured (1)

This question looks at enzymes and enzyme regulation. It is important to be aware of how enzymes are regulated. Short-term regulation can be changes in substrate or product conformation, or changes in enzyme conformation (allosteric regulation, phosphorylation, proteolysis). Long-term regulation involves changes in rate of protein synthesis or degradation.

Enzyme cascades involve initial enzyme signals being geometrically amplified very quickly. This can involve phosphorylation or proteolysis and is important clinically when thinking about mechanisms of blood clotting.

3.
   a. Autosomal recessive disorder (1)
   b. 100% (1)
   c. Cystic fibrosis transmembrane conductance regulator (CFTR) (1)
   Any one of the following scores one mark: total of two marks.
   Lung infections
   Meconium ileus
   Pancreatitis
   Malabsorption
   Infertility
   d. Newborn screening via immunoreactive trypsinogen (1)
   e. Any one of the following scores half a mark: total of two marks
   Respiratory signs – cough, wheezing, breathlessness

Gastrointestinal signs – foul-smelling, greasy stools, poor weight gain and growth, severe constipation

f. Due to blockage of airways as a result of mucus build-up, decreased mucociliary clearance and inflammation (1)

g. The proportion of individuals carrying a particular variant of a gene that also expresses an associated phenotype (1)

This case study is based on cystic fibrosis, which is an autosomal recessive disease caused by mutation in the CFTR gene on Chromosome 7. CFTR is an ATP-responsive chloride channel that is found in epithelial cells of multiple organs, responsible for moving chloride ions out of an epithelial cell to the mucus, thereby playing a critical role in fluid and electrolyte balance across epithelial tissues. Sodium ions follow the chloride ions therefore resulting in movement of water out of the cell. Hence, defective CFTR leads to decreased secretion of chloride and increased reabsorption of sodium and water, which ultimately results in thicker mucus, promoting infection and inflammation.

Signs and symptoms can be grouped by the organ affected. Typically, CF affects the respiratory tract (chronic/recurrent cough, recurrent infections, haemoptysis, dyspnoea), gastrointestinal tract (meconium ileus, failure to thrive, pancreatic insufficiency, malabsorption) and urogenital tract (infertility, amenorrhea).

Cystic fibrosis is a common exam question that can be incorporated into any question type, whether it is based on genetic inheritance or clinical. An in-depth knowledge of this condition would be a necessity.

4.

a. X-linked recessive (1)

b. The high mutation rates in DMD reflect the fact that the dystrophin gene is one of the longest human genes, therefore provides a bigger target for mutagenic agents (1)

c. This is known as germline mosaicism therefore mutations in the egg cell (½) or mutations in the sperm cell (½)
Mutations in egg cell: 8–9% (½)
Mutations in sperm cell: 8–9% (½)

d. One mark for each muscle type identified along with any of the associated histological feature: total of three marks

Muscle type	Histological feature
Skeletal	Striated Peripherally located nuclei Multi-nucleated
Smooth	Non-striated Centrally located nuclei Spindle-shaped cells
Cardiac	Striated Centrally located nuclei Branching cells

   e. Any three of the following score one mark:
     CK, LDH, myoglobin, troponin, AST.
   f. Catalyses reaction from creatine + ATP to phosphocreatine + ADP (1)

            CK

     Creatine + ATP <---> phosphocreatine + ADP

     This reaction is reversible therefore ATP can be generated from
     phosphocreatine and ADP. This is important in tissues and cells that
     rapidly consume ATP as phosphocreatine serves as an energy reservoir
     for the rapid regeneration of ATP (1)

DMD is a common question topic when looking at the theme of genetic inheritance. Knowledge of the processes of mitosis and meiosis underpin this area.

DMD is a condition where no dystrophin is produced. Dystrophin is a protein that plays an important role in sarcolemma stability. Therefore it typically presents with progressive proximal muscular dystrophy with distinctive pseudohypertrophy of the calves. Gait abnormality is also common. Be aware of other muscular dystrophy conditions especially Becker's muscular dystrophy where there is abnormal dystrophin. Practise drawing and interpreting pedigrees as these are common as well.

  5. Any one of the following scores half a mark: total of one mark
    a. Blood loss, for example, menorrhagia or GI bleeding
      Poor diet
      Malabsorption, for example, celiac disease
    b. Occurs within the red bone marrow (1)
      Any one of the following scores half a mark: total of one mark
      Co-factors – iron, vitamin B12, folate
    c. One mark for labelling axis
      One mark for correct shape of myoglobin and adult haemoglobin

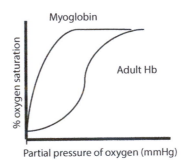

    d. The Hb oxygen dissociation curve shows a sigmoidal shape because it
      contains four globin chains and oxygenation of each chain induces a
      conformational change which increases the affinity of the haem of the
      remaining chains for oxygen (1)
      A myoglobin oxygen dissociation curve shows a hyperbolic shape
      because it contains a single globin chain (1)

e. Any one of the following factors with the effect scores one mark: total of three marks
Please note, students must specify increase or decrease of factor to score marks.
Decrease temperature, increase [H+], decrease pCO_2, decrease red cell 2,3 DPG level all causes a right shift in the curve indicating decreased oxygen affinity, that is, higher P50 value.
Increase temperature, decrease [H+], increase pCO_2, increase red cell 2,3 DPG level all cause a left shift in the curve indicating increased oxygen affinity, that is, lower P50 value.

This question concentrated on the oxygen dissociation curve, which shows the saturation of haemoglobin at various partial pressures of oxygen thereby showing the equilibrium of oxyhaemoglobin and non-bonded haemoglobin at various partial pressures. At high partial pressures haemoglobin binds to oxygen and when the blood is fully saturated, all red blood cells are in the form of oxyhaemoglobin. The partial pressure of oxygen decreases as red cells travel to areas of tissue that lack oxygen and hence oxyhaemoglobin releases oxygen to form haemoglobin.

The sigmoid shape of this curve is due to the co-operative binding of oxygen to the four polypeptide chains of haemoglobin.

Be aware of all the different factors that can affect oxygen binding and different oxygen curves for both foetal haemoglobin and myoglobin.

6.
   a. Case band is heavier (1) because higher molecular weight proteins move more slowly through the gel than lower molecular weight proteins (1)
   b. 110 base pairs, (1) because the mutated strip would not be cut by the restriction enzyme (1)
   c. Tropocollagen consists of a triple helix. The key property is the ability of tropocollagen to spontaneously self-assemble into collagen fibrils (1) which offers great strength and stability via covalent cross-links (1)
   d. The principal bone salt that provides rigidity and strength to bones and teeth (1)
   e. Osteoblasts (1)
   f. Chondrocytes (1)
   g. Elastic cartilage (1)

This question is based on techniques used in molecular genetics.

The methods used here are protein electrophoresis and restriction enzymes. Proteins are charged molecules and will move towards the anode or the cathode when placed within an electric field. Therefore proteins can be separated on the basis of size, shape or charge. SDS is an anionic surfactant hence applies a negative charge to the protein. An electric field is applied and causes the negatively charged proteins to migrate across the gel away from the negative electrode. Depending on the size, small molecules fit easily through the pores in the gel hence travel further down the gel while larger molecules remain near the point of origin.

Be aware of other techniques that are used and their uses, for example, analysis of DNA at the gene level can be via Southern hybridisation.

7.
  a. Autosomal recessive (1)
  b. Adenine to thymine (1)
     Glutamic acid to valine (1)
  c. Dad – BB^s (½)
     Mum – BB (½)
  d. Total of three marks for correct diagram.

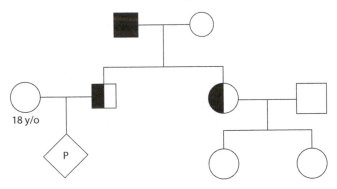

  e. 50% (1)
  f. Any one of the following in each section scores one mark: total of two marks.
     i. Worry of knowing about diseased state and possible treatments required unnecessarily from a very young age
        Potential prejudice in personal or professional life
     ii. Decision to abort foetus
        Burden of future care and medical treatment

This question is based on patterns of inheritance of gene disorders, which in this case is sickle cell anaemia. This is an autosomal recessive pattern of inheritance where heterozygotes are carriers and homozygotes are affected with the condition.

Sickle cell anaemia is a point mutation in the haemoglobin β-chain which causes the haemoglobin to polymerise under low-oxygen states. The resulting RBC deformity and increased endothelial adherence lead to haemolysis, vaso-occlusive crises and micro-infarcts.

MCQ

1. A

If both the father and son are affected this cannot be either X-linked dominant or recessive as in X-linked dominant a man passes on his Y chromosome to all of his sons and his X chromosome to all of his daughters. Therefore you are only left with options A, B or C. It cannot be C because disorders with mitochondrial inheritance result from mutations in mitochondrial DNA which only females can pass on to their children. The answer can only be A because the stem mentions that the father is affected and in autosomal recessive both parents will be unaffected and carry one copy of the mutated gene (carriers).

2. C

Remember Chargaff's rule states that there is always an equal ratio (1:1) of pyrimidine and purine bases in DNA. Therefore if the total amount of adenine is 23% there must be 23% of thymine. This leaves 54% (100%–46%) to be shared amongst guanine and cytosine, hence 27% each (54% divided by 2).

3. E

A TATA box is a DNA sequence found in the promoter regions of eukaryotic genes. It is a sequence that is located 25–35 base pairs upstream of the transcription site. Typically the TATA box has a core DNA sequence of 5'TATAAA-3'. The TATA binds RNA polymerase II and a series of transcription factors to form an initiation complex. It is necessary for transcription as RNA polymerase II cannot recognise the initiation sites on its own.

4. E

Factors that cause a right shift of the oxygen dissociation curve include increased temperature, decreased pH and increased 2,3 DPG.

Note in chronic anaemia, red cell 2,3 DPG levels rise. Other factors that shift the curve to the right are physiological states where tissues require more oxygen such as during exercise and shock.

5. B

Reverse transcriptase – synthesises cDNA from mRNA template
RNA polymerase – produces RNA from DNA template
Ribonuclease III (RNase III) – cuts pre-miRNA transforming it into miRNA

6. E

Compound heterozygosity is the presence of two different mutated recessive alleles at a particular locus that can cause genetic disease in a heterozygous state.

Examples of genetic diseases include phenylketonuria, Tay–Sachs disease, sickle cell syndrome and cystic fibrosis.

7. F

Chromosome inversions occur when a chromosome breaks in two places and the resulting piece of DNA is reversed and reinserted into the chromosome. Inversions can be classed into pericentric or paracentric. Pericentric inversions involve the centromere whereas paracentric inversions do not involve the centromere.

Be aware of all types of chromosomal rearrangement that can occur , for example, deletions, duplications, inversions and translocations.

EMQ

This question is based on the topic of blood clotting cascade.

8. G

Von Willebrand disease is the most common hereditary coagulation abnormality. This case classically describes this condition with symptoms of excessive bleeding following a tooth extraction, easy bruising and increased menstrual flow. Haemophilia can be distinguished here as it usually presents with haemarthrosis with a normal PT and prolonged APTT. Disseminated intravascular coagulation will show a prolonged PT and APTT.

9. C

The coagulation cascade is divided into the extrinsic and intrinsic pathway. The extrinsic pathway begins in the vessel wall where damaged endothelial cells release tissue factor and activate factor VII. This complex then activates factor X. The intrinsic pathway begins in the bloodstream where factor XII is activated by vascular surface changes. Both pathways meet at the final common pathway.

10. F

This case describes pulmonary embolism (PE). When clinically assessing the risk of PE the patient must show breathlessness and/or tachypnoea with or without other symptoms such as pleuritic chest pain or haemoptysis. If the patient presents with this, does the patient have absence of another explanation for these symptoms or is there a presence of a major risk factor (e.g. recent major surgery, previous DVT/PE)? If the answer to these is yes it is considered a high probability of PE. In this case with the information provided we consider this as an intermediate probability and hence D dimers are checked which are raised. In this situation we would start LMWH and request radiological imaging.

Body Tissues (Chapter 2)

1.
   a. Labelling of each correct element scores one mark: total of three marks.

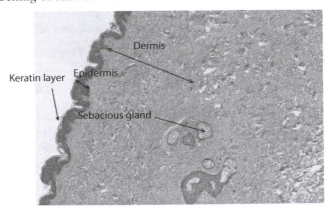

b. Epidermal stem cells reside in the basal layer of the epidermis and divide to give rise to transient amplifying cells, (1) which further divide and differentiate as they migrate through the stratum spinosum, stratum granulosum and finally reaching the stratum corneum. (1) The keratino-cytes in the stratum corneum are named corneocytes and this indicates the completion of the differentiation of keratinocytes. These cells will eventually shed off through desquamation (1)

c. Basal cell carcinoma (½)
Squamous cell carcinoma (½)

d. UV radiation (1)

e. UV radiation penetrates the skin causing damage to the skin's cellular DNA and producing genetic mutations that can lead to skin cancers (1)

f. Any two of the following scores one mark:
Lymphatic system
Haematogenous
Transcoelomic

2.

a. Labelling of each correct element scores half a mark: total of two marks.

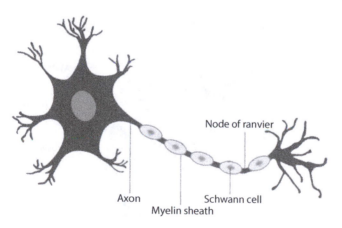

b. Schwann cells form the myelin around myelinated peripheral axons (1) allowing the conduction of local flow of current to the next node of Ranvier, thus the action potential leaps from node to node enhancing its velocity (saltatory conduction) (1)

c. Any one of the following scores one mark: total of two marks.
Astrocytes: Maintain a chemical environment for neuronal signalling
Oligodendrocytes: Provide support and insulation to axons
Microglial cells: Scavenger cells that remove cellular debris from sites of injury or normal cell turnover
Ependymal cells: Production of cerebrospinal fluid

d. Wallerian degeneration is the process that results when the axon separated from the neuron's cell body degenerates distal to the injury (1) as a consequence of the severed axon. The process occurs in the distal axon stump usually after 24–36 hours of the injury followed by a process of regeneration (1)

e. Neuropraxia, axonotmesis, neurotmesis (1)

f. 90 days (1)

This question focuses on both the central and peripheral nervous systems. It is important to appreciate the differences between these systems and the different types of cells involved despite having similar actions within the two systems.

Wallerian degeneration is a key concept that occurs both in the central (CNS) and peripheral nervous system (PNS). However, there are key differences that occur between the two systems. In the PNS, degeneration is initiated by macrophages which remove the myelin and axonal debris. The Schwann cells then guide regeneration of axons from existing stumps at a rate of approximately 1mm/day. In the CNS, axonal regeneration is much slower as it takes approximately 2–4 weeks for macrophages to remove the myelin debris. This is because the debris contains inhibitory factors which slow the regeneration process. Astrocytes then proliferate into the transfected area forming astrocytic scars that block the pathways for axonal growth.

3.

a. Labelling of each correct element scores half a mark: total of two marks.

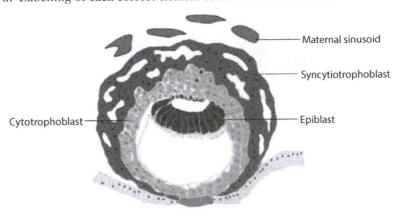

b. Implantation occurs on the posterosuperior wall of the uterus (1) and is completed by the 10th–11th day following fertilisation (1)

c. Due to abnormal persistence of primitive streak tissue (1)

d. Endoderm, mesoderm, ectoderm (1)

e. The neural tube is formed by a process called neurulation. This process begins with the formation of a neural plate, a thickening of the ectoderm. (1) The two dorsolateral apical surfaces of the neural folds meet, fuse at the dorsal midline and separate from the overlying ectoderm, which is now referred to as the neural crest. (1) Forces generated by the surface epithelium as it expands towards the dorsal midline cause elevation of the neural folds causing closure of the neural tube (1)

f. Any one of the following scores one mark:
Spina bifida
Anencephaly
Encephalocele
Hydranencephaly
Iniencephaly

This question looks at human embryogenesis. The basis of embryogenesis starts with the germinal stage (fertilisation, cleavage, blastulation, implantation, embryonic disc) followed by gastrulation and neurulation. It is also important to read about the basic concepts of organogenesis.

In this particular question the scenario was based on a sacrococcygeal teratoma. This is a tumour that is located at the coccyx and derived from the primitive streak. The majority of these tumours are benign and usually discovered via an elevated alpha-fetoprotein at 16 weeks of pregnancy, or by ultrasound which shows an enlarged uterus often due to polyhydramnios.

4.
a. Correct labelling of element (1)

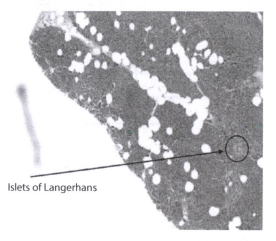

Islets of Langerhans

b. Any one of the following scores one mark: total of two marks
Islets of Langerhans: Glucagon, insulin, somatostatin, amylin, pancreatic polypeptide, ghrelin
c. Merocrine involves the secretion of that cell via exocytosis (1) from secretory cells and deliver their content into extracellular space (1) Examples include the pancreas, sweat glands and salivary glands (1)
d. Each correct answer scores half a mark; total of two marks

Gonad	Both
Adrenal	Endocrine
Parathyroid	Endocrine
Goblet cell	Exocrine

e. The sphincter of Oddi is a muscular valve that controls the flow of bile and pancreatic juice (digestive juices) through ducts from the liver and pancreas into the duodenum. (1) When this becomes dysfunctional (e.g. due to stenosis) the sphincter fails to relax causing the back-up of digestive juices thereby causing pancreatitis (1)

This question is based on the function of the pancreas, as it is one of the very few organs that have both endocrine and exocrine functions. In relation to the pancreas, pancreatitis is a common exam topic and good knowledge will be required. The most common causes of acute pancreatitis are gallstones, ethanol and trauma. The pathogenesis of acute pancreatitis involves cellular injury, for example, via gallstones which then lead to deleterious effects such as the activation of trypsinogen to trypsin thereby triggering the zymogen activation cascade. Patients typically complain of sudden severe epigastric pain that radiates to the back. Investigations will show a raised serum amylase (around three-fold the upper limit of normal) and a form of imaging will be required, for example, ultrasound or CT scan.

5.

   a. Labelling of each correct element scores half a mark: total of three marks.

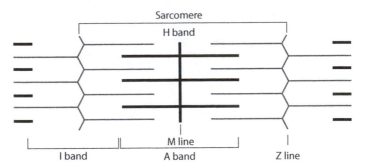

   b. A band: Myosin (½)
      I band: Actin (½)
   c. The motor nerve stimulates an action potential to pass down a neuron to the neuromuscular junction. At the neuromuscular junction, acetylcholine vesicles are released, which bind to the receptor on the sarcolemma causing sodium influx into the muscle fibre, generating an action potential within the muscle fibre. (1) The action potential travels through the T-tubules allowing calcium channels to open and release calcium into the cytoplasm. (1) Calcium activates the actin–myosin binding sites and cross bridges between the actin and myosin heads via ATP. (1) Relaxation occurs when calcium it pumped back into the sarcoplasmic reticulum, breaking the link between actin and myosin (1)
   d. Cardiac muscles are incapable of regeneration (1) so following damage, fibroblasts invade and lay down scar tissue (1)

This question focuses on one of the muscle types, striated muscle. However, it is important to be able to compare the properties of the various muscles. Below is a table which compares skeletal, cardiac and smooth muscle.

	Skeletal	Cardiac	Smooth
Fibre appearance	Striated	Striated	Non-striated
Cell shape	Elongated	Branching	Spindle shaped
Contraction	Voluntary	Involuntary	Involuntary
Nuclei	Multiple, peripherally located	Single, centrally located	Single, centrally located

6.

    a. Labelling of each correct element scores one mark: total of two marks.

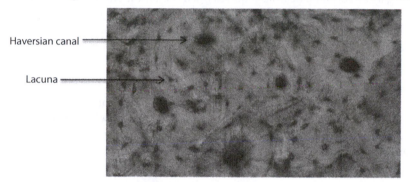

Haversian canal

Lacuna

Reproduced with permission of Dr Ana Gonzalez & Prof Giles Perryer

    b. Oestrogen levels decrease rapidly when women reach menopause. (1) Oestrogen has a protective effective on bone by reducing bone resorption and increasing bone formation, therefore decreased levels will increase the risk of osteoporosis (1)

    c. Any one of the following scores half a mark: total of one mark.
       Age
       Low body mass (<19 kg/m^2)/anorexia nervosa
       Family history of hip fracture
       Past history of hip fracture
       Corticosteroid therapy
       Smoking
       Alcohol

    d. Any one of the following scores one mark:
       Bisphosphonates
       Human monoclonal antibody

    e. Fracture healing can be divided into three stages:
       i. Reactive: A haematoma forms at the fracture site and inflammatory exudation from ruptured blood vessels initiate an inflammatory response (1)

    ii. Reparative: Periosteal cells proximal to the fracture gap develop into chondroblasts which form hyaline cartilage. Periosteal cells distal to the fracture gap develop into osteoblasts which form woven bone. Ingrowth of capillaries into the callus and increased vascularity follow (1)
Hard callus formation: Replacement of woven bone with lamellar bone via endochondral ossification. This lamellar bone is known as trabecular bone (1)

    iii. Remodelling: The trabecular bone is resorbed by osteoclasts followed by deposition of compact bone via osteoblasts (1)

This question looks at fracture healing, which occurs either by direct intramembranous or indirect healing. These consist of both intramembranous and endochondral bone formation. The most common pathway is indirect healing as direct bone healing requires open reduction and internal fixation. Indirect healing follows a specific pathway involving an acute inflammatory response, recruitment of mesenchymal stem cells to generate a primary cartilaginous callus, followed by revascularisation and calcification, and finally remodelling to restore normal bone structure.

Osteoporosis is one of many bone conditions. Diagnosis is via a DEXA scan which measures the bone density and a T score of <-2.5 confirms osteoporosis. Management is centred on preventing fragility fractures, which include lifestyle advice, nutrition, exercise and smoking cessation. Medication includes bisphosphonates (first line), denosumab, strontium ranelate, raloxifene and calcium and vitamin D supplements.

MCQ

1.B

Options A, D and E are not related to bone formation, therefore the answer can only be either B or C. There are two major processes that create bone during embryonic development. Endochondral ossification is a process that uses hyaline cartilage as the model for long bone formation. Intramembranous ossification is a process that uses mesenchyme tissue in the development of flat bones.

2. A

Haematoxylin is a basic dye that stains dark blue/violet when bound to acidic structures. Eosin is an acidic dye that stains red/pink when bound to basic structures. Options B, C, D and E are all basic structures. Examples of acidic structures include DNA in the nucleus and RNA in ribosomes and in the rough endoplasmic reticulum.

3. D

Epithelium can be classified as either simple or stratified. Simple squamous epithelium is found in locations where rapid diffusion or filtration occurs, for example, the glomerulus of the kidney and alveoli in the lungs. Simple cuboidal epithelium lines the surface of small excretory ducts of organs and glands, for example, salivary glands. Simple columnar epithelium are found throughout the body's organs in areas that are highly secretive or absorptive, for example, small intestine. Pseudostratified epithelium is usually confined to the larger respiratory airways of the nasal cavity, trachea and bronchi. Transitional epithelium are found in tissues that stretch, for example, the lining of the bladder and urethra. Goblet cells are associated with simple columnar epithelium of the gastrointestinal tract.

4. B

Both the omental bursa and the greater omentum are derived from the dorsal mesogastrium, which is the mesentery of the stomach region.

The dorsal mesoduodenum is the mesentery in the area of the duodenum, which disappears later thereby leaving the duodenum and pancreas to lie retroperitoneally. The ventral mesentery forms the falciform ligament, ligamentum teres and lesser omentum. The dorsal mesocolon is the mesentery of the hindgut (splenic flexure, descending and pelvic colons, rectum and anal canal).

5. D

There are three main types of arteries: elastic, muscular and arterioles. Elastic arteries receive blood directly from the heart. Muscular arteries distribute blood to various parts of the body, for example, femoral artery. These arteries have a distinguishing characteristic of both internal and external layers. The internal elastic layer is between the tunica intima and tunica media. The external elastic layer is between the tunica media and tunica adventitia. Arterioles are small arteries that deliver blood to capillaries. Capillaries are thin-walled vessels that allow gas exchange. Venules are small branches of veins.

6. E

The epidermis is divided into five layers: stratum basale, stratum spinosum, stratum granulosum, stratum lucidum and stratum corneum. The stratum basale contains the dividing cells (keratinocytes). The cells in the stratum spinosum are spiny shaped. The cells in the stratum granulosum contain keratohyalin granules. The stratum lucidum is a layer that only occurs in certain hairless parts of the body namely the palms of the hands and the soles of the feet. The stratum corneum is the outermost layer. The keratinocytes in this layer are called corneocytes and contain no nucleus.

7. C

The lymphatic capillary within a villus of the small intestine is a lacteal.

The Crypt of Lieberkuhn is a gland found in the epithelium lining the small and large intestine. Plicae circulares is a projection into the lumen of the small intestine. Brunner's glands are located in the duodenum protecting it from the acidic chyme. Peyer's patches are nodules of lymphatic cells that are found in the ileum.

EMQ

This question is based on the various different cells associated with the different types of epithelium

8. A

Squamous alveolar cells are also known as type I pneumocytes. These cells are involved in the process of gas exchange between the alveoli and blood.

9. J

Clara cells are found in the ciliated simple epithelium which secrete glycosaminoglycans to protect the bronchiole lining.

10. D

Type II pneumocytes are involved in the secretion of pulmonary surfactant which decreases the surface tension within the alveoli. Infant respiratory distress syndrome is caused by developmental insufficiency of pulmonary surfactant production.

Metabolism (Chapter 3)

1.
 a. 4.0–6.0 mmol/L (1)
 b. i. ≥ 7.0 mmol/L (½)
    ii. ≥ 11.1 mmol/L (½)
 c. Increase glycogen synthesis in liver and muscle (1)
    Increase glucose uptake in muscle and adipose by GLUT4 (1)
    Decrease production of glucose by inhibiting glycogenolysis in the liver (1)
    Decrease production of glucose by inhibiting glyconeogenesis primarily in the liver (1)
 d. Half a mark for each correct curve: total of one mark

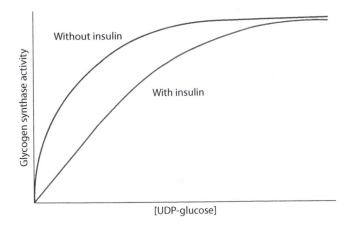

    f. HbA1c is formed in a non-enzymatic glycation pathway by haemoglobin's exposure to plasma glucose. (1) This test is limited to an average over three months because the lifespan of red blood is 120 days (1)

    g. Fructosamine (1)

This question focuses on diabetes. Blood sugar levels in diagnosing diabetes are different dependent on the plasma glucose test. In a random glucose test or a 2-hour postprandial test, a level of 11.1 mmol/L is diagnostic whereas a fasting glucose test level of 7.0 mmol/L or more is diagnostic. Insulin is a hormone that has many physiological effects not only on carbohydrate metabolism but also lipid (increases lipogenesis and decreases lipolysis) and protein (increases protein synthesis and decreases protein degradation) metabolism. Enzyme kinetics is a common exam topic and it is important to appreciate that a competitive inhibitor increases K_m but has no effect on V_{max}; an uncompetitive inhibitor decreases both K_m and V_{max}; a non-competitive inhibitor has no effect on K_m but decreases V_{max}.

In patients with diseases that reduce red blood cell lifespan, for example, haemolytic anaemia, sickle cell anaemia, thalassemia, HbA1c may be misleadingly low. Therefore fructosamine can be used to monitor blood sugar levels. This involves the glycated fraction of all plasma proteins but predominantly albumin, and reflects average glucose levels over the previous 2 weeks.

  2.

    a. Any one of the following scores one mark.

       Corneal arcus

       Tendon xanthoma

       Xanthelasma

    b. Any one of the following scores one mark: total of two marks.

       Premature coronary heart disease

       Stroke

       Heart attack at early stage

       Aortic aneurysm

    c. Cholesterol molecules orient themselves in the bilayer with their hydroxyl groups close to the polar head groups of phospholipid molecules, which results in the lipid bilayer becoming less deformable. (1) It acts as a buffer, preventing lower temperatures from inhibiting fluidity and preventing higher temperatures from increasing fluidity (1)

    d. Any one of the following scores one mark: total of two marks.

       Used as a precursor by testis, ovaries or adrenal gland for the synthesis of steroid hormones

       Used as a precursor for the synthesis of vitamin D

       Used as a precursor in the synthesis of bile acids

    e. LDL particle binds to LDL receptor (½)

       LDL receptors cluster in clathrin-coated pits (½)

       Coated pits pinch off to form endocytic vesicles and are uncoated (½)

       Vesicles are directed towards endosome where the presence of low pH causes conformational change of LDL receptors leading to release of LDL (½)

LDL particles are delivered to lysosomes and degraded releasing cholesterol (½)

LDL receptors return to plasma membrane and the cycle repeats (½)

This question focuses on the topic of cholesterol. Cholesterol is essential in maintaining membrane structural integrity and fluidity. The physiology of cholesterol in terms of its function, biosynthesis and transport is important. In terms of synthesis, this is via the mevalonate pathway where HMG-CoA reductase is the rate-limiting enzyme and this is important, as a group of medication called statins inhibits this enzyme thereby lowering cholesterol levels. Cholesterol is transported within lipoproteins, which consist of chylomicrons, VLDL, IDL, LDL and HDL.

3.
   a. Low T4: Antibodies which block the TSH receptors or attack and slowly destroy cells of the thyroid gland therefore causing reduced secretion of T4 (1)

      High TSH: Low T4 gives a positive feedback response in the hypothalamus and anterior pituitary gland, which stimulates more TRH and TSH release, respectively (1)

      Diagnosis: Hypothyroidism (1)
   b. Iodine deficiency (1)
   c. TSH can give trophic effect to cause hypertrophy, hyperplasia and increase vascularity in the thyroid gland (2)
   d. In follicular cells (1)
   e. T3 has a very short half-life while the half-life of T4 is much longer, ensuring a steady supply of T3 (1)
   f. Labelling of each correct element scores one mark: total of two marks. The colloid is the place where thyroid hormones are stored.

      The follicle is labelled for reference only.

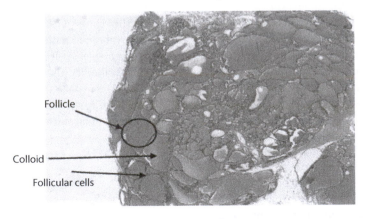

This question focuses on the thyroid gland with relation to hypothyroidism. It is important to note the pathways involved in thyroid function in terms of the hypothalamic-pituitary-thyroid axis. The hypothalamus secretes TRH that stimulates production of TSH from the anterior pituitary. TSH increases the production and release of T4 and T3 from the thyroid then exerts negative feedback on TSH production. It is the basis of this understanding that will help you in the diagnosis of the various thyroid conditions.

	TSH	T4	T3
Hypothyroidism	Increase	Decrease	–
Subclinical hypothyroidism	Increase	Normal	–
Hyperthyroidism	Decrease	Increase	Increase
Subclinical hyperthyroidism	Decrease	Normal	Normal
Central hypothyroidism (hypothalamic or pituitary disorder)	Decrease	Decrease	–
Sick euthyroidism	Decrease	Decrease	Decrease

4.
   a. Any one of the following scores half a mark: total of three marks.
      Protein: Provides energy and essential amino acids
      Fat: Provides energy and essential fatty acids
      Water: Maintains hydration
      Vitamins and minerals: Prevents signs and symptoms of deficit state
      Carbohydrates: Provide energy for the body's activities
      Fibre: Necessary for normal GI function
   b. 12,000 kJ (1)
   c. Any two of the following scores one mark: all three for two marks.
      Basal metabolic rate
      Exercise
      Diet induced thermogenesis
   d. Energy input greater than energy expended (1)
   e. Due to high glycogen stores in the liver (1)
   f. Any one of the following scores half a mark: total of two marks.
      Hypertension
      Osteoarthritis
      Type 2 diabetes
      Coronary artery disease
      Stroke
      Cancer, for example, colon

This question gives an overview of nutrient metabolism. Metabolism is the processes which derive energy and raw materials from food stuffs and using them to support repair, growth and activity of the tissues of the body. Metabolism involves both catabolism (breakdown of large molecules to release energy) and anabolism (uses energy to make molecules for growth and maintenance). If expenditure exceeds intake, energy stores will deplete then other body components (primarily protein) will be utilised to provide energy.

5.
   a. Excess alcohol intake leads to an increase in the ratio of NADH:NAD+ The build-up of NADH inhibits gluconeogenesis leading to hypoglycaemia (1)
   A lowered NAD+:NADH ratio leads to accumulation of acetaldehyde which causes damage to the liver (1)
   b. K_m is defined as the substrate concentration that gives half maximal velocity of an enzymatic reaction (1)
   In high alcohol levels the microsomal ethanol oxidising system (MEOS) converts ethanol to acetaldehyde and MEOS has high K_m but low affinity (1)
   c. Increased bilirubin levels – jaundice (1)
   Inhibition of oxidation of fatty acids causing an accumulation of triglycerides causing a fatty liver – usually asymptomatic (1)
   d. Any two of the following symptoms scores one mark and one mark for its explanation.
   Autonomic: sweating, anxiety, hunger, tremor, palpitations, dizziness
   Hypoglycaemia provokes an autonomic response causing increased release of adrenaline and noradrenaline.
   Neuroglycopenic: confusion, drowsiness, visual trouble, seizures, behaviour changes, slurred speech
   Due to lack of glucose for functioning of the CNS – glycopenia
   e. Any two of the following for two marks:
   Dietician
   Alcoholics anonymous
   Meals on wheels
   General practitioner
   Psychotherapist
   Family therapy, for example, Al-Anon

This question focuses on alcohol metabolism and its effects. Alcohol is primarily metabolised through alcohol dehydrogenase (ADH) which oxidises alcohol to acetaldehyde in the cytosol which is further oxidised by acetaldehyde dehydrogenase to acetate in the mitochondria. Acetaldehyde is a toxic metabolite in the blood and the NADH produced from the reaction is used for ATP generation through oxidative phosphorylation. Acetate is converted to acetyl-CoA and oxidised in the TCA cycle. A microsomal ethanol oxidising system consists of cytochrome P450 which has a high K_m but low affinity for alcohol in chronic alcoholism, whereas ADH has low K_m but high affinity for alcohol in low alcohol levels.

The effects of alcohol primarily stem from the generation of NADH which increases the NADH:NAD+ ratio in the liver. Consequently, fatty acid oxidation is inhibited, inhibits gluconeogenesis and increases production of lactate. Therefore, this may result in lactic acidosis, alcohol-induced liver disease and hypoglycaemia.

6.
   a. Any one of the following scores one mark: total of two marks.
      Dehydration
      Tachypnoea
      Deep breathing (Kussmaul respiration)
      Ketotic breath
   b. i. <400 ml/day (1)
      ii. >3 L/day (1)
   c. A ketone body produced in the liver which can be used by the brain as a source of energy (1)
      Insulin deficiency and a rise in stress hormones therefore a fall in the insulin:glucagon ratio which results in increased ketogenesis (1)
   d. A compensatory reaction where bicarbonate is used to react with ketoacids to achieve a normal pH (1)
   e. Increased glycogenolysis (1)
      Increased gluconeogenesis (1)
      Increased ketogenesis (1)

This question focuses on diabetic ketoacidosis (DKA), which is a high anion gap metabolic acidosis due to an excessive blood concentration of ketone bodies. The most common precipitating factor for DKA is infection. DKA occurs as a result of insulin deficiency together with excess stress hormone release. The absence of insulin results in decreased glucose uptake peripherally by muscle and fat. Excess stress hormone causes the mobilisation of free fatty acids from fat cells and a switch in hepatic lipid metabolism to ketogenesis. In addition, hyperglycaemia and ketonaemia causes an osmotic diuresis with dehydration and loss of electrolytes.

7.
   a. Cushing's syndrome (1)
   b. Any of the explanations below with two associated signs or symptoms scores two marks.
      Excess production of cortisol causing increased androgen production leading to central obesity, moon face, hirsutism, sexual dysfunction, amenorrhea/oligomenorrhoea
      Excess production of cortisol causing glycogenolysis leading to hyperglycaemia
      Excess production of cortisol causing loss of collagen leading to purple striae around abdomen, thighs, buttocks
   c. Hypernatraemia (½)
      Hypokalaemia (½)
   d. Because the mineral corticoid receptor binds both aldosterone and cortisol with equal affinity (1)
   e. Corticotropin releasing factor from the hypothalamus (1) causes the release of ACTH from the anterior pituitary gland, which acts on the adrenal cortex causing release of cortisol (1)

    f. Small cell carcinoma of the lung is derived from bronchial neuroendocrine cells, which naturally have secretory functions. (1) Upon malignant transformation, these cells already have the basic metabolism to secrete various hormonal agents (1) and require less perturbation of their DNA to release inappropriate agents (1)

This question looks at the condition, Cushing's syndrome. The clinical features associated with this condition stem from the excess cortisol production, which leads to glycogenolysis, increased vascular sensitivity to catecholamine, increased androgen production, increased aldosterone and proteolysis. The main cause is glucocorticoid therapy. Other causes include ACTH-secreting pituitary adenoma (Cushing's disease), ectopic ACTH production, for example, from small-cell lung cancer and carcinoid tumours. Diagnosis is based on a raised plasma cortisol followed by localisation of the source. This can be determined through other tests such as the dexamethasone suppression test, plasma ACTH level and appropriate imaging studies.

8.
    a. Any one of the following scores one mark: total of two marks.
      Diffuse thickening of the appendicular wall
      Mucosal haemorrhage
      Purulent exudate
    b. Any one of the following scores one mark: total of two marks.
      Transmural infiltration of polymorphs
      Mucosal ulceration
      Local fibrinopurulent peritonitis
      Vascular thrombosis
    c. Any one of the following for half a mark: total of one mark.
      Prostaglandin E2
      Interleukins (IL-1, IL-6)
    d. This is because the amount of glucose filtered exceeds the capacity of the kidney tubules to reabsorb glucose, which results in glucose in the urine. Glucose draws water into the urine by osmosis (1)
    e. Insulin requirements need to be increased (1) as infection causes a stress response which increases counter regulatory hormones to insulin therefore increasing blood sugar levels (1)
    f. In the liver: Inhibition of gluconeogenesis and glycolysis (1)
      In the muscle: Glycogen synthesis (1)

This question focuses on diabetes, which is classified as type I (autoimmune destruction of insulin-secreting pancreatic beta cells) or type II (reduced insulin secretion and/or increased insulin resistance). There are various insulin regimens but commonly a biphasic regimen, either four times a day or once daily. It is important that patients are aware of adjusting doses according to finger prick glucose test, exercise, illness and calorie intake.

9.
   a. Graves' disease (1)
   b. Thyrotropin-releasing hormone from the hypothalamus (1) stimulates the production of TSH from the anterior pituitary. (1) TSH increases production and release of thyroxine (T_4) and triiodothyronine (T_3) from the thyroid which exerts negative feedback on TSH production (1)
   c. Increased cell metabolism (1)
      Increased catecholamine effect (1)
   d. Recurrent laryngeal nerve (1)
      Parathyroid gland (1)
      Superior laryngeal nerve (1)
      Carotid artery (1)

This question focuses on hyperthyroidism. This is commonly caused by Grave's disease which is due to circulating IgG autoantibodies that bind to and activate G protein-coupled thyrotropin receptors. Other causes include toxic multinodular goitre, and toxic adenoma. In particular thyroid eye disease is seen in 25%–50% of people with Grave's disease, which may be the first presenting sign of Graves' disease. Features may include exophthalmos, proptosis, papilloedema and ophthalmoplegia.

The physiological effects of thyroxine include increasing cell metabolism via nuclear receptors and therefore are key for growth and mental development.

MCQ

1. D

This patient is likely to have De Quervain's thyroiditis which commonly occurs after a viral infection. Patients usually present with fever, and sudden painful thyroid enlargement with the disease subsiding within 6–8 weeks. Option A will does not routinely cause hyperthyroidism. Options B and C are causes of hyperthyroidism but toxic multinodular goitre is usually seen in the elderly and Graves' disease does not usually settle without treatment. Option E can cause hyperthyroidism but is usually painless.

2. B

Glycogen phosphorylase catalyses the rate-limiting step in glycogenolysis. This process is regulated by glucagon (stimulates) and insulin (inhibits).

Option A is inhibited by phosphorylation and activated by the binding of citrate. Option C is allosterically inhibited by ATP and ADP, and activated by glucose 6-phosphate. Option D is indirectly stimulated by insulin and indirectly inhibited by glucagon. Option E is activated by fructose 1,6-biphosphate and inactivated by ATP.

3. A

Insulinoma is diagnosed by fasting hypoglycaemia (<2.5 mmol/L) associated with an elevated insulin level. Proinsulin, C-peptide and insulin are all increased.

4. C

Glutamate plays an important role in disposal of excess nitrogen by undergoing deamination. Ammonia is then excreted as urea. Glycine predominantly acts as a precursor to proteins such as in the formation of collagen. Aspartate is used in the biosynthesis of proteins and is produced from oxaloacetate. Lysine is also used in synthesis of proteins and is metabolised to produce acetyl-CoA. Tyrosine occurs in proteins that are part of signal transduction processes.

5. D

This patient is likely to have Marfan syndrome, which is a disorder that affects connective tissue. This condition is an autosomal dominant disorder caused by mutations in the FBN1 gene that encodes fibrillin-1.

6. B

Hyperlipidaemia can be classified into different types according to lipid profile. Type I is characterised by increased chylomicrons, type IIa is characterised by increased LDL, type IIB is characterised by increased LDL and VLDL, type III is characterised by increased IDL, type IV is characterised by increased VLDL and finally type V is characterised by increased chylomicrons and VLDL.

7. A

This patient is likely to be suffering from hypothyroidism, which usually shows an elevated TSH and low T_4. TSH levels usually increase before serum T_4 or T_3 therefore TSH measurement would be the most sensitive test in diagnosing hypothyroidism.

EMQ

This question is based on various metabolic disorders and associated molecules.

8. D

This patient is likely to be suffering from glycose-6-phosphate dehydrogenase (G6PD) deficiency. G6PD is an enzyme in the pentose phosphate pathway, involved in maintaining adequate amounts of NADPH in cells which maintains levels of glutathione.

9. G

Glycolysis converts glucose into pyruvate. The energy yield from this process is two ATP and two NADH. Four regulatory enzymes are involved in glycolysis which include hexokinase, glucokinase, phosphofructokinase and pyruvate kinase of which phosphofructokinase-1 is the rate-limiting enzyme.

10. C

This patient is likely to be suffering from phenylketonuria which results from the absence of phenylalanine hydroxylase. This enzyme converts phenylalanine to tyrosine. High levels of phenylalanine lead to the production of neurotoxic by-products (phenylpyruvic acid and phenylethylamine). This condition usually presents with progressive developmental delay and general learning disability. Some other signs and symptoms include seizures, recurrent vomiting and severe behavioural disturbance.

Membranes and Receptors (Chapter 4)

1.
   a. cAMP – Protein kinase A (1)
      cGMP – Protein kinase G (1)
      Diacylglycerol – Protein kinase C (1)
      Ca^{2+} = Ca^{2+}/calmodulin-dependent protein kinase (1)
   b. The increase in intracellular calcium following an action potential reaches the synaptic terminal and binds to synaptotagmin. (1) This causes a conformational change in the protein complex, bringing the vesicle closer to the membrane and transmitter release through the fusion core created by the SNARE complex (1)
   c. Removal of neurotransmitters can be either through degradation (½) or reuptake (½).
   d. i. Acetylcholine (1)
      ii. Noradrenaline (1)
   e. Atropine acts on sweat glands causing anhydrosis (½)
      Atropine has no effect on vascular smooth muscle (½)

This question focuses on effector mechanisms in intracellular signalling, particularly second messengers. Some important generating effects include adenylyl cyclase and phospholipase C. Adenylyl cyclase is a plasma membrane protein that can be activated (via G_s) or inhibited (via G_i) by activation of different receptors. This enzyme hydrolyses cellular ATP to produce cyclic AMP, which interacts with protein kinase A therefore phosphorylating other proteins and their subsequent effects. Phospholipase C involves the hydrolysis of PIP_2 to generate IP_3 and DAG. IP_3 interacts with intracellular receptors on the endoplasmic reticulum to allow efflux of Ca^{2+} into the cytoplasm. DAG interacts with protein kinase C causing protein phosphorylation.

2.
   a. Acetylcholine (½) acting on M2 muscarinic receptors (½)
   b. Second messengers – inositol trisphosphate (IP_3) and diacylglycerol (DAG) (1)
      IP_3 interacts with specific intracellular receptors on the endoplasmic reticulum (ER) to allow calcium to leave the lumen of the ER and enter the cytoplasm (1)
      DAG activates protein kinase C which in turn activates proteins inside the cell by phosphorylation (1)

c. One mark for correct shape of graph
One mark for each correct labelled channel point with their action: total of three marks

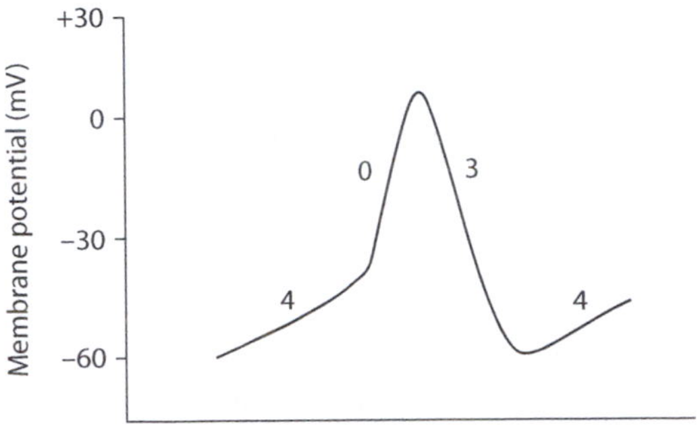

4 = 'Funny' channel – Influx of slow Na^+ ions causing depolarization
0 = L-type Ca^{2+} channel – increased Ca^{2+} conductance through L-type Ca^{2+} channel causing further depolarization
3 = K^+ channel – Efflux of K^+ ions causing repolarization

d. At rest parasympathetic impulses along the vagus nerves slow down the depolarisation of the SA node (1)
e. SA node, AV node, Bundle of His, bundle branches, Purkinje fibres (1)

This questions focuses on the cardiac conduction system. The SA node is the natural pacemaker of the heart. The SA node releases electrical stimuli at a regular rate which passes through the myocardial cells producing contractions which spread through both atria. The stimulus from the SA node (situated in the right atrium) eventually reaches the AV node (situated between the two atria), which in turn travels through the Bundle of His, divides into the left and right bundle branches and through the Purkinje fibres, which causes the ventricles to contract.

3.

a. Chronic alcoholism causes damage to hepatocytes releasing reactive oxygen species and inducing the activation of hepatic stellate cells. (1) Subsequent liver injury causes apoptosis of hepatocytes which contributes to tissue inflammation, fibrogenesis and cirrhosis (1)
b. Disulfiram is an irreversible inhibitor of aldehyde dehydrogenase therefore causing an increase in acetaldehyde concentration, which is responsible for the unpleasant effects of alcohol (1)
c. Alcohol dehydrogenase (½)
Aldehyde dehydrogenase (½)
d. Any one of the following scores one mark: total of two marks.
Age
Gender
Impaired liver or kidney function
Pharmacogenetics
Polymorphism

    e. Highest potency – A (½)
       Lowest efficacy – C (½)
    f. This is because it possesses low intrinsic activity despite having a high affinity for its receptor. (1) This is a description of a partial agonist.
    g. Non-linear kinetics is when increases in drug exposure are not linearly related to increases in dose administered. (1) Therefore, when consuming alcohol once the maximum elimination capacity is reached there is no further elimination hence drug clearance decreases with increasing alcohol concentration (1)

This question is based on drugs and receptors. Agonists are drugs that have both affinity and efficacy whereas antagonists have affinity only. The equilibrium dissociation constant (K_d) is a measure of affinity where the lower the value, the higher the affinity. The effective concentration giving 50% of the maximal response (EC_{50}) is a measure of potency. It is often the case that EC_{50} is less than K_d and not all receptors are required to be occupied to get a maximal response. This is because the relationship between receptor occupancy and response is non-linear. Some tissues have more receptors than required to produce a maximum response, that is, spare receptors. These receptors increase sensitivity which allows responses at low concentrations of agonist.

  4.
    a. The red blood cell cytoskeleton is a network of spectrin and actin molecules. (1) Spectrin forms long, flexible heterodimers through lateral associations with alpha and beta subunits that in turn associate head-to-head to form a heterotetramer of $\alpha_2\beta_2$ (1)
    b. Biconcave (1)
    c. Any of the following scores half a mark: total of one mark.
       Myocardial infarction
       Liver disease
       Pulmonary embolism
       Tumour necrosis
       Cerebrovascular accident (stroke)
    d. LDH converts pyruvate to lactate (1)
       Producing lactate regenerates NAD^+ and allows glycolysis to continue (1)
    e. Any one of the following scores one mark:
       Bilirubin
       Haptoglobin
       Reticulocytes
       Full blood count
    f. The increase in reticulocytes reflects the attempt to compensate for the blood loss (1)
    g. Any one of the following scores one mark: total of two marks.
       Abdominal pain
       Dyspnoea
       Weakness
       Light headedness

This question focuses on membrane proteins and the cytoskeleton. Biological membranes are composed of a lipid bilayer with associated membrane proteins, which may be integral or peripheral. The erythrocyte cytoskeleton is important in maintaining the deformability necessary for erythrocytes to travel through capillary beds without lysis. Hereditary spherocytosis is a condition where spectrin levels are depleted and cells become less resistant to lysis cleared by the spleen. The shortened survival of red blood cells and inability of the bone marrow to compensate leads to haemolytic anaemia.

5.
  a. Myelin sheath (1)
  b. Loss of myelin sheath causes a decrease in membrane resistance (1) and decreased length constant (1) and therefore insufficient current to generate an action potential as it reaches the next node of Ranvier (1)
  c. Delayed visual evoked potential (1)
  d. One mark for correct labelled axis
     One mark for correct shape of graph

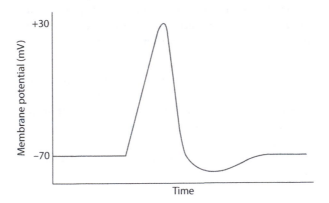

  e. Depolarisation – due to influx of sodium ions (1)
     Repolarization – due to efflux of potassium ions (1)
     Refractory phase – due to inactive conformation of sodium channels (1)

This question focuses on the action potential and conduction of nervous impulse. Action potentials depend on ionic gradients and relative permeability, and only occur once a threshold is reached. Once a certain membrane potential is reached a positive feedback occurs as sodium channels begin to open. Repolarization of action potential occurs due to inactivation of sodium channels and activation of potassium channels. After an action potential, most of the sodium channels have been inactivated and require time to recover before they open again.

A change in membrane potential in part of an axon can spread to adjacent areas of the axon and occurs due to the spread of local current. The further the local current spreads down the axon, the faster the conduction velocity of the axon. A high membrane resistance, a low membrane capacitance and a large axon diameter will all lead to a high conduction velocity.

6.
   a. Any of the following scores one mark:
   Legionella pneumophila
   Chlamydophila species
   Pneumocystis jiroveci
   b. Any of the following scores half a mark: total of four marks.

Synapse	Neurotransmitter	Receptor
a	Acetylcholine	Nicotinic acetylcholine
b	Noradrenaline	Beta-2 adrenergic
c	Acetylcholine	Nicotinic acetylcholine
d	Acetylcholine	M_3 muscarinic

   c. Bronchoconstriction (1)
   Increased secretion from submucosal glands (1)
   Vasodilation of pulmonary blood vessels (1)
   d. Parasympathetic – cyclic GMP (1)
   Sympathetic – cyclic AMP (1)

This questions focuses on the autonomic nervous system. The parasympathetic nervous system regulates organ and gland functions during rest. The preganglionic nerve releases acetylcholine at the ganglion acting on nicotinic acetylcholine receptors of the postganglionic neurons. The postganglionic nerve releases acetylcholine stimulating muscarinic receptors of the target organs. The sympathetic nervous system maintains internal organ homeostasis and initiates the stress response. The preganglionic nerve releases acetylcholine at the ganglion acting on nicotinic acetylcholine receptors of the postganglionic neurons. The postganglionic nerve releases noradrenaline activating adrenergic receptors of the target organs. However, two exceptions are the sweat glands and chromaffin cells of the adrenal medulla. Postganglionic sweat glands release activating muscarinic receptors. Preganglionic neurons synapse directly with chromaffin cells with stimulation release of noradrenaline and adrenaline.

MCQ

1. D

The resting membrane potential for a ventricular myocyte is about –90 mV. The resting potential for nerve cells is about –50 to –70 mV and –20 to –30 mV for animal cells. The resting membrane potential for heart SA node is –55 to –60 mV and –90 to –100 mV for skeletal muscle.

2. A

There are three main groups of ion channels which are voltage gated channels, extracellular ligand activated channels and intracellular ligand gated ion channels. Examples of voltage gated channels include sodium, potassium and calcium. Examples of extracellular ligand gated ion channels include nicotinic acetylcholine receptors, GABA and ROMK channel. Example of intracellular ligated ion channels includes CFTR.

3. C

Tyrosine kinase receptors are cell surface receptors for growth factors, cytokines and hormones. Examples of tyrosine kinase receptors include epidermal growth factor receptor, fibroblast growth factor receptor, insulin receptor and vascular endothelial growth factor receptor. GABA receptors are either ligand gated ion channel or g protein-coupled receptors, dependent on the subtype.

4. A

Oxaloacetate competes with the substrate for binding at the active site of succinate dehydrogenase therefore it is a competitive inhibitor. A non-competitive inhibitor binds at a site distinct from the active site. An irreversible inhibitor inactivates an enzyme by bonding covalently to a particular group at the active site. Allosteric inhibition is when a substrate binds to an enzyme other than the active site.

5. E

This scenario describes the condition of myasthenia gravis, which is an autoimmune condition mediated by antibodies to nicotinic acetylcholine receptors at the junction between the nerve and muscle. Option A describes the condition Lambert-Eaton. Option B describes the condition multiple sclerosis. Option D describes the Tolosa–Hunt syndrome.

6. B

Parasympathetic nerve supply arises through three main areas which include the cranial nerves, vagus nerve and pelvic splanchnic nerve. Other options all arise from a sympathetic nerve.

7. C

Phase I metabolism involves modification and this can be via oxidation, reduction or hydrolysis. Phase II metabolism involves conjugation making the metabolite more water-soluble therefore facilitating excretion as well as decreasing pharmacological activity. This can be achieved through, for example, methylation, sulfation, acetylation or glucuronidation.

EMQ

This question is based on effector mechanisms in intracellular signalling.

8. G

IP3 exerts its effects by interacting with specific intracellular receptors on the ER to allow calcium to leave the lumen of ER and enter the cytoplasm. This will result in the activation of calcium-sensitive protein kinases.

9. E

Protein kinase A activity is dependent on cellular levels of cyclic AMP.

10. J

Phosphorylase kinase activates glycogen phosphorylase to release glucose-1-phosphate from glycogen. Glycogen phosphorylase can be activated by glucagon, adrenaline, protein kinase A and calmodulin.

Mechanism of Pathology (Chapter 5)

1.
   a. Hyperplasia – increase in tissue or organ size due to increase in number of cells (1)
   b. Immune (½)
      Inflammatory (½)
   c. Lymphomas are disorders caused by malignant proliferations of lymphocytes (1)
      Hodgkin's lymphoma (½)
      Non-Hodgkin's lymphoma (½)
   d. Apoptosis – programmed cell death of individual cells (1)
      Necrosis – death of a contiguous group of cells in response to injury (1)
      Differences: apoptosis is an active process and a non-inflammatory reaction (1) whereas necrosis is a passive process and an inflammatory reaction (1)
   e. Staging – extent of spread of a cancer (1)
      Any one of the following scores half a mark: total of one mark.
      Size of tumour
      Node status
      Distant metastasis

This question focuses on cell injury (reversible or irreversible), which occurs as a consequence of hypoxia. In reversible cases ischaemia occurs, leading to decreased oxidative phosphorylation in the mitochondria resulting in decreased ATP. The principal effect is a decrease in sodium pumps and increased glycolysis. In irreversible cases the injurious agent causes an increase in cytosolic calcium which leads to events such as decreased ATP, decreased phospholipids and nuclear chromatin damage.

Be aware of the various types of necrosis and key differences between necrosis and apoptosis.

2.
   a. Any one of the following scores half a mark: total of two marks.
      Redness
      Heat
      Swelling
      Pain
      Loss of function

b. Any one of the following scores one mark: total of two marks
Histamine: vascular dilatation and transient increase in vascular permeability
Prostaglandins: potentiate the increase in vascular permeability
Leukotrienes: increase in vascular permeability and emigration of neutrophils
Cytokines: increase in vascular permeability and emigration of neutrophils
c. Bacteraemia causes release of toxins (½). The subsequent release of inflammatory mediators causes an inflammatory response (½). This leads to widespread vasodilation (½) through the action of nitric oxide. Unresponsiveness or depletion of vasoactive factors leads to hypotension (½).
d. Any one of the following scores half a mark: total of one mark.
Temperature <36°C or >38°C
Heart rate >90 bpm
Respiratory rate >20 breaths per minute
WBC <4 × 10⁹/L or >12 × 10⁹/L
e. Illustrating layers of gram-positive organisms (1)
Illustrating layers of gram-negative organisms (1)
Gram-positive organisms have a thicker peptidoglycan layer in their cell walls which retains the crystal violet in gram staining (1)

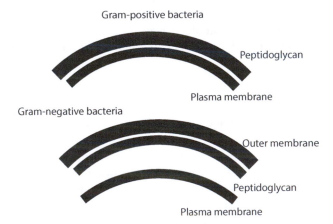

Gram-positive bacteria

Peptidoglycan

Plasma membrane

Gram-negative bacteria

Outer membrane

Peptidoglycan

Plasma membrane

This question focuses on acute inflammation. Acute inflammation is a response of living tissue to injury of short duration. This process typically involves a vascular reaction (accumulation of fluid exudate and neutrophils), which is controlled by a variety of chemical mediators and is usually a protective mechanism but may lead to local complications and systemic effects. Changes in vascular flow involve transient vasoconstriction of arterioles followed by vasodilatation and increased permeability of blood vessels. The resulting stasis causes margination of neutrophils, which then result in rolling, adhesion and emigration of neutrophils. Finally, neutrophil chemotaxis and phagocytosis occurs.

3.

a. Any one of the following scores one mark: total of three marks:

Benign	Malignant
Nuclear variation in size and shape is minimal	Nuclear variation in size and shape minimal to marked
Diploid	Range of ploidy
Low mitotic count, normal mitosis	Low to high mitotic count, abnormal mitosis
Retention of specialisation	Loss of specialisation
Structural differentiation retained	Structural differentiation shows wide range of changes
Organised	Not organised
Non-invasive	Invasive
Slow growing	Fast growing

b. Colon contents are more liquid in the ascending colon, and so disturbance of bowel habit is less likely (1)

c. Any one of the following categories with an example scores one mark: total of two marks
   Receptor tyrosine kinase – epidermal growth factor receptor, vascular endothelial growth factor
   Regulatory GTPases – Ras protein
   Transcription factor – Myc

d. Any one of the following with an example scores one mark: total of two marks
   Radiation – ultraviolet, ionising
   Chemicals – polycyclic aromatic hydrocarbons, aromatic amines, nitrosamines
   Viruses – hepatitis B, Epstein–Barr, human papilloma

e. Screening every 2 years to all men and women aged 60–75 (1) by using faecal occult blood home testing kits (1)

This question focuses on neoplasia. Neoplasia is defined as abnormal growth of cells which persists after the initiating stimulus has been removed, and this can either be benign or malignant. The ability of cells to break through the basement membrane and spread is characteristic of malignant cells. The occurrence of tumours can be thought due to an accumulation of genetic alterations. Both intrinsic and extrinsic factors can contribute to the development of cancer. Intrinsic factors include age, immune factors, hormones and inheritance whereas extrinsic factors include radiation, chemicals and viruses.

4.

a. Inflammation (½) – hematoma formation and inflammatory exudation from ruptured blood vessels
   Soft callus formation (½) – growth of callus forming woven bone
   Hard callus formation (½) – replacement of woven bone by lamellar bone
   Remodelling (½) – substitutes trabecular bone with compact bone

    b. Any one of the following scores one mark: total of two marks.
First intention healing: opposed wound edges, less scarring, less
contraction, repair time shorter
Second intention healing: larger scar, more late contraction to reduce
volume defect, repair time longer

    c. Any one of the following scores half a mark: total of one mark.
Fibroblasts
Myofibroblasts
Macrophages
Endothelial cells

    d. Any one of the following scores one mark: all three for two marks.
Hemodynamic changes (stasis, turbulence) – alterations in normal
blood flow
Endothelial injury – irritation of the vessel
Hypercoagulability – alterations in constitution of blood

    e. Any one of the following scores half a mark: total of one mark.
Local – blood supply, infection, foreign material, radiation damage
Systemic – age, drugs, specific dietary deficiency, general state of health,
general cardiovascular status

    f. LMWH is typically shorter than 18 units therefore accelerates the
bridging of antithrombin with factor Xa only, and not thrombin. UFH
is larger than 18 units therefore inhibits the function of thrombin as
well as factor Xa (1)
LMWH has a shorter polymer therefore does not bind proteins readily, therefore no monitoring is required but UFH has an unpredictable
anticoagulant effect due to long polysaccharide bind to plasma protein,
therefore requires monitoring (1)

This question focuses on the topic of repair and regeneration. Labile cells
(e.g. epithelial cells) or stable cells (e.g. hepatocytes) are able to regenerate whereas
permanent cells (e.g. neurons) are unable to divide or regenerate. Fibrous repair
occurs through three main mechanisms: 1) cell migration, 2) angiogenesis and 3)
extracellular matrix production and remodelling. Healing by primary intention
occurs with apposed wound edges. There is minimal clot and granulation, and
the epidermis is able to regenerate. Healing by secondary intention occurs in
unopposed wound edges and the clot dries forming an eschar. However, with this
healing the repair process produces much more granulation tissue.

MCQ

1. C

Enzymes released from acute pancreatitis damage the surrounding fat by the
production of soaps. The damaged pancreas releases lipase and amylase as
markers. Coagulative necrosis involves protein denaturation and liquefactive
necrosis involves enzyme release. Caseous necrosis is most often encountered in
tuberculosis infection.

2. B

This case describes Barrett's oesophagus which is characterised by replacement of stratified squamous epithelium lining the oesophagus with simple columnar epithelium with goblet cells. This is a process of metaplasia.

3. E

A fatty streak is the first macroscopic feature of atheroma formation. It involves lipid deposits in the intima. This may be the precursor to simple and complicated plaques. Microscopic features include proliferation of smooth muscle, accumulation of foam cells, extracellular lipid, fibrosis, necrosis and cholesterol clefts.

4. A

The suture is recognised as a foreign body, therefore recruiting macrophages that are activated and transformed into foreign body giant cells.

5. B

Malignant neoplasm can be characterised by uncontrolled growth of cells and spreading of cells into surrounding tissue and spread to distant sites. Pleomorphism can occur in both malignant and benign neoplasms although more commonly in malignant. An increased nuclear/cytoplasmic ratio is a feature of malignancy but is not the best indicator: invasion into surrounding tissue suggests malignancy more.

6. E

This case describes tuberculosis which is a granulomatous inflammatory disease. A granuloma consists of epithelioid macrophages, which fuse together to form a giant cell.

7. D

Cell cycle progression is controlled by two key checkpoints, which are G_1 and G_2. Cells are least sensitive when in the S phase, followed by G_1, G_2 and the most sensitive being M phase. Therefore the most sensitive to radiation would be the second checkpoint (G_2/M) which results in chromosomal abnormalities in mitosis.

EMQ

This question is based on the topic of cell injury.

8. I

Hemosiderin staining is the appearance of a brownish patches under the skin that occurs as a by-product of the breakdown of red blood cells.

9. G

Reperfusion injury occurs when blood supply returns to the tissue after a period of ischaemia. The restoration of circulation during a period of hypoxia leads to inflammation and oxidative damage through the production of reactive oxygen species.

10. A

The diagnosis of myocardium infarction rests on the presence of necrotic myocardium with the earliest finding being hypereosinophilia. Later there is infiltration of neutrophils with apoptosis. As it progresses, coagulative necrosis is established.

Infection and Immunity (Chapter 6)

1.
   a. An X-linked agammaglobulinaemia (inherited immunodeficiency disease) (1)
   b. Mutations in the gene coding for Bruton tyrosine kinase (1)
   c. Intravenous infusion of immunoglobulin (1)
   d. Active immunisation (½)
      Passive immunisation (½)
   e. Any of the following scores half a mark: total of one mark.
      Active immunisation: vaccinia, rotavirus, polio, yellow fever, BCG, typhoid, pertussis, meningococcus, pneumococcus
      Passive immunisation: diphtheria, hepatitis A, hepatitis B, measles (rubella), rabies, tetanus, varicella zoster virus
   f. Passive immunity from mother (1)
   g. IgA deficiency (1)
   h. DiGeorge syndrome (1)
      Severe combined immunodeficiency (1)
      Chronic granulomatous disease (1)

This question focuses on immunodeficiency. Immunodeficiency can be classified as either primary or secondary. Primary immunodeficiency is relatively rare, congenital or acquired and is usually due to an intrinsic defect. Secondary immunodeficiency is relatively common, acquired and usually secondary to other conditions. The resulting effect from immunodeficiency may affect T or B cells, antibody production, phagocytic cells, complement or other immune components. You should always suspect immunodeficiency in patients who present with severe, persistent, unusual or recurrent infections.

2.
   a. Any of the following scores one mark: total of two marks.
      Bronchitis
      Lung cancer
      Pneumonia
      Bronchiectasis
      Pulmonary embolism
      Heart failure

b. Labelling of each correct element scores half a mark: total of two marks.

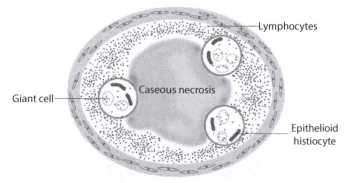

c. Labelling of each correct element scores one mark: total of six marks.

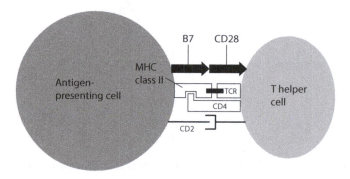

This question focuses on antigen processing and presentation. T cells primarily coordinate and regulate the adaptive immune response, regulate functions of innate effectors and major effectors in recognition and killing of virally infected and tumour cells. However, T cells can be pathogenic, for example, recognition of non-self MHC is a major cause of organ transplant rejection. Antigen processing is a process that prepares antigens for presentation to T lymphocytes. The source of microbial peptides dictates where they are presented to either class I or II MHC molecules. MHC class I molecules then present the antigen to cytotoxic CD8+ T cells which kill the infected cell, whereas MHC class II molecules present the antigen to helper CD4+ T cells which promote adaptive immunity. However, costimulatory signals (B7 and CD28) are required for T-cell activation.

3.

　a. Any three of the following scores one mark:
　　Malnutrition
　　Drug-induced, for example, immunosuppressants, chemotherapy
　　HIV
　　Nephrotic syndrome
　　Burns

Asplenia

Physiological, for example, age, pregnancy

Tumours, for example, lymphoproliferative disease/leukaemia

b. Activation of complement system (1) which leads to opsonisation of the formation of a membrane attack complex

Activation of effector cells (1) which leads to antibodies binding to pathogens causing agglutination

Production of natural antibodies (1) which leads to lysis

c. Labelling of each correct element scores half a mark: total of three marks.

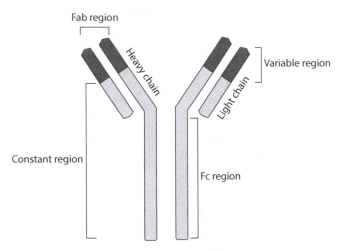

d. Any one of the following scores one mark: total of two marks.

Streptococcus viridians

Enterococci

Staphylococcus aureus

Staphylococcus epidermidis

Any fever, invasive procedures or recreational drug use (1)

This question focuses on an overview of antibodies and the complement system. Antibodies have various functions which include opsonisation of bacteria for phagocytosis (IgM, IgG), neutralisation of bacteria (IgM, IgG), opsonisation of bacteria for complement mediated killing (IgM, IgG), and agglutination of bacteria (IgM). In response to an antigen, the first antibodies produced are IgM. Replicating B cells soon switch to producing IgG (secondary response). This switch in immunoglobulin class involves heavy chain constant region only. The classical pathway is antibody-mediated which results in complement system activation.

4.

a. IgE antibody (1)

b. An extrinsic allergen causes a Th2 response causing B cells to produce IgE antibodies (priming). (1) The IgE antibodies bind to receptors on the surface of mast cells which are now 'sensitised' (sensitisation). (1) Re-exposure to the allergen (elicitation) causes preformed

IgE to trigger release of mediators such as histamine and prostaglandins. (1) These mediators primarily cause vasodilation and smooth-muscle contraction (1)

c. Bronchospasm (1)
Mucosal oedema (1)
Increased mucous secretion (1)

d. Adrenaline: constriction of resistant arterioles on alpha-1 receptors increases blood pressure and relaxes airways via beta-2 receptors (1)
Corticosteroids: suppress allergic immune/inflammatory effect (1)

This question focuses on the topic of hypersensitivity. There are four types of hypersensitivity reaction which are best explained with the table below.

	Mediator	Mechanism	Example
Type I	IgE antibody	Mast cell activation	Anaphylaxis Asthma
Type II	IgG or IgM antibody	Antibody directed against cell surface antigens mediates cell destruction via complement activation	Goodpasture's syndrome Autoimmune haemolytic anaemia
Type III	IgG antibody	Formation of immune complex	Rheumatoid arthritis Serum sickness
Type IV	T cells	Sensitised TH1 cells release cytokines that activate macrophages	Contact dermatitis Tuberculin reaction

5.

a. Lymphocytosis – increase in number of lymphocytes in the blood (1)
Atypical mononuclear cells – lymphocytes with some morphological properties of monocytes (1)
Diagnosis – infective mononucleosis (1)

b. Epstein–Barr virus (1)

c. IgM (1)

d. Ampicillin and amoxicillin causes an itchy maculopapular rash (1)

e. Any one of the following signs with an explanation scores two marks.
Hepatomegaly – On inspiration, palpate from the right iliac fossa and continue upwards towards the costal margin until you feel the edge of the liver.
Splenomegaly – On inspiration, palpate from the right iliac fossa towards the left costal margin until you feel the edge of the spleen.

f. Cytotoxic T cell (CD8+ T cell) (1)
Antigens are degraded into peptides within the cell which are displayed at the surface of the cell nestled within a class I major histocompatibility molecule, which are recognised by CD8+ T cell (1)

This question focuses on the T-cell response to intracellular pathogens.
In general, T-cell activation during viral infections involve four key stages:
(1) Activation of dendritic cells (antigen processing), (2) presentation (presentation of viral peptides via MHC I and MHC II molecules), (3) activation of
T cells, (4) effector phase (killing of infected cells, memory T cells). The type of
anti-microbial response is dependent on the type of pathogen. Below is a table
giving a brief description of the anti-microbial defence.

6.
    a. Upper respiratory tract (1)
    b. Any one of the following scores half a mark: total of one mark.

	Cytosolic pathogens	Intravesicular pathogens	Extracellular pathogens and toxins
Peptides bind to	MHC class I	MHC class II	MHC class II
Presented to	CD8 T cells	CD4 T cells	CD4 T cells
Th response	Th1	Th1	Th2
Effector mechanism	CD8 T cells	Macrophages	B cells/antibodies

       Neisseria meningitidis
       Streptococcus pneumoniae
       Group B streptococcus
       Listeria monocytogenes
    c. i. Cryptococcus neoformans (1)
      ii. Mycobacterium tuberculosis (1)
    d. Empirical antibiotic (Cefotaxime or Ceftriaxone) (1)
    e. Irritation of meninges causing irritation of optic nerve (1)
    f. Either of the following scores one mark:
      Kernig's sign
      Brudzinski's sign
    g. Labelling of each correct element scores one mark: total of three marks

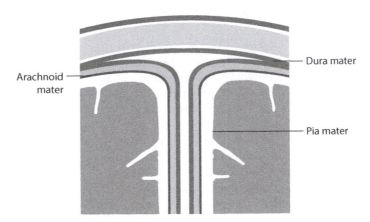

7.

   a. Influenza A (1)

   b. Oseltamivir (1) – Inhibitor of neuraminidase thereby affecting release of viral particles (1)

   c. Active immunisation: involves adaptive immunity where it is induced by inactivated or attenuated live organisms or their products (1)
Passive immunisation: results from the injection of preformed human immunoglobulin (or heterologous antibody) (1)

   d. Any one of the following scores one mark: total of three marks.
Pneumococcal (PCV) vaccine
Rotavirus vaccine
Meningitis B vaccine
5-in-1 vaccine (diphtheria, tetanus, pertussis, polio, haemophilus influenzae type b)

   e. Recombinant DNA-based vaccine (1)

   f. Human immunodeficiency virus (HIV) (½)
Hepatitis C (½)

This question focuses on vaccination. Vaccination aims to prime the adaptive immune system to antigens of a particular microbe so that a first infection induces a secondary response. Active immunisation is given to provide protective responses before people become exposed to a pathogen whereas passive immunisation is given infrequently to people following exposure to a microbe or toxin, or following onset of illness. The main types of antigen include live organisms (natural or attenuated), whole non-living organisms (viruses or bacteria), fragments (viruses or bacterial polysaccharide), toxoids, recombinant DNA-based, adjuvanted and conjugated.

MCQ

1. A

Splitting of C3, into C3a and C3b, by C3 convertase is the control point of the complement system. C3b binds to the surface of pathogens for opsonisation by phagocytes. Factor B is a component of the alternative pathway which binds with C3b, forming a complex that cleaves C5. C6 is part of the membrane attack complex that is involved in cell lysis. Factor H is a complement control protein that regulates the alternative pathway. C5a is a chemotactic factor of the alternative pathway.

2. C

Haemolytic uraemic syndrome (HUS) is most commonly caused by infection with *E. coli* bacteria that produces certain toxins (shiga toxin-producing *E. coli*). Campylobacter, Salmonella and Yersinia are all able to cause bloody diarrhoea but less commonly result in HUS.

3. D

This patient is suffering from hyperacute rejection as a result of incompatibility between donor and recipient blood. Hence preformed antibodies against B antigen will cause agglutination and haemolysis when encountered with erythrocytes with B antigens. Hyperacute rejection occurs within minutes after transplant with destruction of the tissue as a result of preformed antibodies reacting with antigens of the transplanted organ. Acute rejection can occur as early as the first week after transplant with increased risk within the first 3 months and is due to antibody-mediated immunity. Chronic rejection occurs months to years after transplant and is due to the presence of cell-mediated immunity.

4. B

This patient is suffering from tuberculosis (TB). The protective immunity to this infection is cell mediated, causing formation of granulomas. IgE hypersensitivity is involved in allergic reactions. Antibody-mediated immunity and eosinophils are important defences against many bacteria but not the principal defence against TB. Natural killer cells target aberrant cells such as virally infected and tumorigenic cells.

5. D

The following are cell surface markers for particular cells:
CD19 – B lymphocyte
CD3 – T lymphocyte
CD25 – T regulatory cell
CD3 –T helper cell

6. B

A J chain is a protein component of the antibodies IgM and IgA. This chain is expressed by mucosal and glandular plasma cells.

7. E

Upon activation of natural killer (NK) cells, these cells produce a large variety of cytokines and chemokines. All of the options apart from IL-10 are produced by NK cells. IL-10 is primarily produced by monocytes and to a lesser extent lymphocytes and B cells.

EMQ

This question is based on the topic of antibody structure.

8. F

The allotype of an antibody represents the genetically determined differences in antibodies. Most allotypic variation occurs in the constant region of heavy and light chains.

9. H

Antibodies are divided into classes by antigenic determinants on their heavy chains. The Fc region therefore determines the antibody class (or isotype) into IgA, IgD, IgE, IgG or IgM.

10. D

The Fab region of an antibody is responsible for the binding to the antigen whereas the Fc region binds to the Fc receptor on a number of cells, for example, phagocytes, neutrophils and lymphocytes thereby stimulating phagocytosis.

Gastrointestinal System (Chapter 7)

1.
   a. A connection that occurs between the veins of the portal circulation and those of the systemic circulation (1)
   b. Any one of the following scores one mark: total of two marks.
      Portal – left branch of portal vein: systemic superficial veins of anterior abdominal wall
      Portal – superior rectal vein: systemic – middle and inferior rectal vein
      Portal – veins of ascending colon, descending colon, duodenum, pancreas and liver; systemic – renal, lumbar and phrenic veins
      Portal – portal branches in liver; systemic – azygous system of veins above the diaphragm
   c. The underlying liver disease increases the resistance to portal blood flow (1) causing splanchnic vasodilatation with sodium and water retention. (1) This all leads to a significant increase in blood flow through the portal vein (1) which further contributes to portal hypertension and consequent oesophageal varices
   d. Haematocrit level would be normal. (1) This is because haematocrit only falls as extravascular fluid enters the intravascular space to restore volume (1)
   e. The concentration of sodium in isotonic saline solution is similar to that of extracellular fluid (ECF). (1) Therefore, this effectively limits its distribution to the ECF and distributes between the interstitial fluid and plasma (1)

This question focuses on portal hypertension, which is defined as portal venous pressure in excess of 20 mmHg. This results from intrahepatic or extrahepatic portal venous compression or occlusion. Causes include obstruction of portal vein (e.g. thrombosis) or obstruction of flow within the liver (e.g. cirrhosis). Clinical features of portal hypertension include splenomegaly, ascites, spider naevi, caput medusae or oesophageal/rectal varices.

2.
   a. Duodenum – presence of submucosal Brunner's glands (1)
      Ileum – increase in amount of lymphoid tissue of Peyer's patches (1)
      Jejunum – villi are longer and more finger-like and there is absence of Brunner's glands and Peyer's patches (1)

b. If the terminal ileum is damaged, there is malabsorption of bile acids (1), which leads to bile salt deficiency resulting in impaired fat solubilisation (1)

c. The terminal ileum absorbs vitamin B12 therefore malabsorption occurs as it is damaged. (1) Vitamin B12 is a cofactor for DNA synthesis therefore resulting in decreased DNA synthesis in the erythrocyte, hence macrocytosis (1)

d. A high level of bilirubin in plasma causes yellowing of the sclera, skin or mucosae (1)
Increased breakdown of red blood cells results in increased serum bilirubin (unconjugated). (1) This bilirubin is water insoluble therefore cannot be excreted in urine. Intestinal bacteria converts the bilirubin into urobilinogen which is reabsorbed and excreted by the kidneys resulting in increased urinary urobilinogen (1)

This question focuses on the small intestine, which extends from the pylorus of the stomach to the ileocaecal junction. It consists of three parts – the duodenum, jejunum and ileum. The duodenum is the most proximal part of the small intestine and can be divided into four parts (superior, descending, inferior, ascending). The jejunum and ileum are the distal parts of the small intestine. Certain features allow these two parts to be distinguished which is important when undertaking surgery. Some features of the jejunum include red in colour, thick intestinal wall, long vasa recta and fewer arcades. The ileum is pink in colour and has a thin intestinal wall, shorter vasa recta and more arcades.

3.
a. Lateral to inferior epigastric vessel (1)
Pass through internal inguinal ring (1)

b. Herniation of a part of the abdominal viscera through the oesophageal opening of the diaphragm (1)

c. External spermatic fascia (½) – derived from the aponeurosis of the external oblique muscle (½)
Cremaster muscle and fascia (½) – derived from internal oblique muscle and its fascial coverings (½)

d. Internal spermatic fascia (½) – derived from the transversalis fascia (½)

e. During 6th week, the growth of the primary intestinal loop is very rapid and the liver is also growing rapidly. (1) The abdominal cavity is too small to accommodate both so the intestines herniate into the umbilical cord (1)

f. A reflex contraction of the internal oblique and transversus abdominis muscles in response to increased abdominal pressure, (1) which causes the inguinal ring to close like a sphincter around the spermatic cord, protecting against herniation (1)

This question focuses on hernia. There are various types of hernias but inguinal hernias (indirect and direct) are the commonest type. Indirect hernias pass through the internal inguinal ring whereas direct hernias push their way through the posterior wall of the inguinal canal, into a defect in the abdominal wall (Hesselbach's triangle). Indirect hernias lie lateral to the inferior epigastric vessels but indirect hernias lie medial to the inferior epigastric vessels. Two important landmarks are the deep (internal) ring which is at the mid-point of the inguinal ligament and the superficial (external ring) which is a split in the external oblique aponeurosis superior and medial to the pubic tubercle.

4.
   a. Visceral pain caused by distension, inflammation or ischaemia to the abdominal organ localises depending on the embryologic origin. (1) The stomach and proximal half of duodenum are foregut structures and hence peptic ulcer disease causes epigastric pain (1)
   b. Any one of the following scores half a mark: total of one mark.
      Gastrin
      Histamine
      Acetylcholine
   c. Perforation (½)
      Haemorrhage (½)
      Gastric outlet obstruction (½)
      Penetration (½)
   d. Any one of the following scores half a mark: total of two marks.
      Pancreas
      Left suprarenal gland
      Upper pole of left kidney
      Diaphragm
      Spleen
   e. Any one of the following scores one mark: total of two marks.
      Proton pump inhibitors (e.g. omeprazole) – inhibits the ability of parietal cells to produce gastric acid.
      Antibiotics – used to treat ulcers caused by helicobacter pylori infection.
      H_2 antagonists (e.g. ranitidine) – antagonise H_2 histamine receptors on the surface of parietal cells in the stomach thereby decreasing acid secretion.
   f. Gram negative (1)

This question focuses on peptic ulcer disease, which can be classified into duodenal ulcer or gastric ulcer. A duodenal ulcer is far more common than a gastric ulcer with 90% of cases related to helicobacter pylori. A gastric ulcer occurs mainly in the elderly, on the lesser curve. Complications include bleeding, perforation, malignancy and decrease in gastric outflow. Treatments include lifestyle (e.g. reducing alcohol intake and avoiding aggravating foods), helicobacter eradication (triple therapy), drugs to reduce acid (e.g. proton pump inhibitors and H_2 blockers) and stopping any drugs that induce ulcers (e.g. NSAIDs).

5.
   a. Any one of the following scores half a mark: total of one mark.
      Crohn's disease – skip lesions, strictures, aphthous ulcer
      Ulcerative colitis – continuous lesions, mucosa shows erythema and friability
   b. Any one of the following scores half a mark: total of one mark.
      Crohn's disease – transmural inflammation, granulomas
      Ulcerative colitis – mucosal/submucosal inflammation, crypt abscess

c. Any one of the following scores half a mark: total of one mark.
   Erythema nodosum
   Pyoderma gangrenosum
   Aphthous stomatitis
   Anal fissures
   Enterocutaneous fistula
d. Malabsorption of vitamins (K, B1, B2 and B12) (1)
   Watery stools/diarrhoea (1)
e. Any one of the following scores half a mark: total of one mark.
   Perforation
   Massive haemorrhage
   Toxic dilatation
   Failed medical therapy
f. Labelling of each correct element scores one mark: total of four marks.

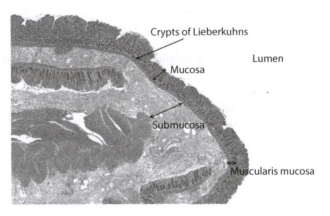

This question focuses on inflammatory bowel disease. The table below highlights the main differences between ulcerative colitis and Crohn's disease.

	Ulcerative colitis	**Crohn's disease**
Age	15–25 years old 55–65 years old	15–30 years old 50–70 years old
Site	Colon especially rectum	From mouth to anus especially terminal ileum
Diarrhoea	Majority	Frequent
Bleeding	Frequent	Variable
Pain	Variable	Frequent
Endoscopy	Mucosa inflammed Contact bleeding	Mucosa inflammed/normal Aphthous ulcers
Histology	Mucosal inflammation Goblet cell depletion Crypt abscess Superficial ulceration	Transmural inflammation Deep ulceration Granuloma

6.
   a. Post-hepatic jaundice (1)
   b. On ingestion of food, cholecystokinin (CCK) is released from mucosa of the duodenum. (1) CCK stimulates contraction of the gallbladder and relaxation of the sphincter of Oddi (1)
   c. Failure to emulsify fats and absence of bile pigment (stercobilinogen) due to obstruction of bile secretion cause pale stools (steatorrhoea) (1) Conjugated bilirubin is reabsorbed into, and filtered in, the kidney causing dark urine due to post-hepatic obstruction (1)
   d. Bile acids, produced in hepatocytes from cholesterol, are conjugated then excreted into bile. (1) Conjugated bile salts are then reabsorbed in the terminal ileum (95%) and returned to the liver by the hepatic portal vein. (1) The remaining bile salts are lost in the faeces (1)
   e. Glucuronyltransferase (1)
   f. Steatorrhoea (bulky, difficult to flush, foul-smelling, oily) (1)

This question focuses on jaundice, which is classified as pre-hepatic, hepatic or post-hepatic. Pre-hepatic jaundice is due to excessive haemolysis where the liver is unable to cope with the excess bilirubin. Findings include unconjugated hyperbilirubinaemia, reticulocytosis, anaemia, increased LDH and decreased haptoglobin. Hepatic jaundice is due to deranged hepatocyte function which may show mixed unconjugated and conjugated hyperbilirubinaemia, increased liver enzymes and abnormal clotting. Post-hepatic jaundice is due to obstruction of the biliary system where passage of conjugated bilirubin is blocked. Findings will show conjugated hyperbilirubinaemia, dark urine and an increase in ALP.

7.
   a. Approximately 6.7 litres (1)
      Saliva (1 litre), pancreatic (1 litre), bile (1 litre), gastric (1.5 litres), small intestine (2 litres), large intestine (200ml) (1)
   b. Metabolic alkalosis (1) – prolonged vomiting causes loss of hydrochloric acid and produces an increase of bicarbonate in the plasma to compensate for the lost chloride. Renal excretion of potassium increases in order to preserve sodium causing hypochloraemic, hypokalaemic metabolic alkalosis (1)
   c. The thirst centre (hypothalamus) has a very high threshold for activation and is only activated by hypertonic plasma. (1) Prolonged vomiting results in hypertonic fluid loss causing hypotonic plasma (1)
   d. Striated muscle in the upper third, striated and smooth muscle in the middle third and smooth muscle in the lower third (1)
   e. Cervical constriction – due to cricoid cartilage at level of C5/6 (1)
      Thoracic constriction – due to aortic arch at level of T4/5 (1)
      Abdominal constriction – at oesophageal hiatus at T10/11 (1)

This question focuses on elements of the thirst mechanism. The thirst centre is situated in the hypothalamus. Antidiuretic hormone (ADH) plays an important role in the maintenance of fluid balance and is secreted by the hypothalamus when plasma osmolality increases. However, the osmotic threshold for thirst is set higher compared to ADH. Four major stimuli to thirst are hypertonicity, hypovalaemia, hypotension and angiotensin II.

8.
   a. Men – 21 units (½)
      Women – 14 units (½)
   b. Presence of regenerating nodules of hepatocytes (½)
      Presence of fibrosis (½)
   c. Pancreatitis (1)
   d. Amylase (1)
   e. Any one of the following scores half a mark: total of one mark.
      Gallstones
      Trauma
      Steroids
      Mumps
      Autoimmune
      Scorpion stings
      Hyperlipidaemia/hypercalcaemia
      ERCP
      Drugs, for example, azathioprine
   f. Liver disease (cirrhosis) causes a decrease in bile salt synthesis, leading to impaired absorption and vitamin K deficiency (1)
   g. Chronic pancreatitis causes extensive scaring and destruction of the pancreatic tissue. (1) Diabetes results from the destruction of insulin-producing cells (1)
   h. Precontemplation, contemplation, preparation, action, maintenance (2)

This question focuses on pancreatitis, which is a condition characterised by an inflammatory process caused by effects of enzymes released from pancreatic acini. The pathogenesis underlying acute pancreatitis involves duct obstruction, acinar damage (from reflux or drugs) and enzyme release (protease, lipase, elastase). Chronic pancreatitis is a chronic inflammatory condition that involves parenchymal destruction, fibrosis, loss of acini and duct stenosis.

9.
   a. Visceral peritoneum is supplied by non-somatic nerves therefore visceral pain is poorly localised, diffuse and vague (1)
   b. Any three correct answers scores one mark: all correct answers score two marks.
      A – right gastric artery
      B – left gastric artery
      C – short gastric artery
      D – left gastroepiploic artery
      E – right gastroepiploic artery
   c. Haematogenous (1)
      Transcoelomic (1)
   d. The blood supply of the gastrointestinal tract drains directly through the liver (1)

e. Any one of the following scores one mark: total of two marks.
Ach released by parasympathetic neurons
Gastrin secreted by G cells
Histamine released by mast cells

f. When the pH of the stomach gets too low, this stimulates delta cells to release somatostatin (1) which acts directly on parietal cells and also inhibits the release of positive regulators histamine and gastrin (1)

This question focuses on the stomach. The control of acid secretion is via three main factors (gastrin, histamine, acetylcholine) that act on the parietal cell to stimulate acid secretion. The export of H^+ ions is via proton pumps from the canaliculi. The phases of control of acid secretion include the cephalic phase, gastric phase and the intestinal phase. The stomach also secretes mucus and bicarbonate for defence; however, these can be breached by alcohol, helicobacter pylori and NSAIDs which will result in peptic ulcers.

10.
a. Epigastric pain is aggravated by eating hence patients avoid eating, therefore there is a loss of appetite and consequent weight loss (1)

b. This produces urease which converts urea to carbon dioxide and ammonia which is a basic molecule and neutralises the acidic environment (1)

c. Gastroduodenal artery – haemorrhage (1)
Pancreas – pancreatitis (1)

d. Microcytic anaemia (1)

e. Any of the following scores one mark:
Iron deficiency anaemia
Thalassaemia
Sideroblastic anaemia

f. Ferritin (½)
Serum iron (½)
Serum transferrin (½)
Total iron binding capacity (½)

g. i. Alkaline mucus produced by prostaglandin E2 forming the unstirred layer (1)
ii. Alkaline secretion from pancreatic juice and bile (1)

This question focuses on peptic ulcer disease but with an emphasis on the duodenum. The duodenum extends 20 to 30 cm from the pyloric sphincter to the ligament of Treitz. The duodenum is divided into four parts: the cap, descending, transverse and ascending portions. The majority of duodenal ulcers occur within 4 cm of pylorus and on the anterior wall of the superior part of the duodenum. If the ulcer penetrates the duodenal wall, duodenal contents may enter the peritoneal cavity resulting in peritonitis. The superior duodenum is in close proximity to the liver, gallbladder and pancreas hence any of these structures may adhere to the inflamed site and become eroded and ulcerated. Posterior penetrating ulcers erode into the pancreas and underlying gastroduodenal artery.

11.
 a. Metaplasia (1)
 b. Stratified squamous to simple columnar (1)
 c. Upper third – inferior thyroid artery (1)
 Middle third – oesophageal branches of the thoracic aorta (1)
 Lower third – left gastric artery (1)
 d. The oesophagus enters the stomach at an acute angle (1)
 The walls of the intra-abdominal section of the oesophagus is compressed when there is a positive intra-abdominal pressure (1)
 The folds of mucosa aid in occluding the lumen at the gastro-oesophageal junction (1)
 The right crus of the diaphragm has a 'pinch-cock' effect (1)
 e. Recurrent laryngeal branch of vagus nerve (1)

This question focuses on the oesophagus. The oesophagus originates at the level of C6 and descends entering the abdomen by piercing the right crus of the diaphragm through the oesophageal hiatus at T10. There are two sphincters (upper and lower) in the oesophagus which act to prevent air entry and reflux of gastric contents. The upper oesophageal sphincter is at the junction between the pharynx and oesophagus. The lower oesophageal sphincter (physiological) is located at the gastro-oesophageal junction.

MCQ

1. C

Bilirubin is the end product of haeme metabolism. Pigment stones are the most frequent type seen in cirrhosis, while cholesterol represents about 15% of all stones. Calcium carbonate and calcium oxalate are commonly found in kidney stones.

2. A

Enteropeptidase converts trypsinogen to trypsin which activates pancreatic enzymes. Chymotrypsin is a component of pancreatic juice acting in the duodenum. Lactase is located in the brush border of the small intestine that hydrolyses the bond between galactose and glucose in lactose. Elastase breaks down elastin in connective tissues. Erepsin is found in the intestinal juices where it digests peptides into amino acids.

3. E

The primary secretion of saliva is isotonic with plasma and its electrolyte composition is similar to plasma. It becomes hypotonic as it travels through the duct. However, upon chewing, for example, the flow rate increases. Substances whose concentrations increase with increased flow rate include sodium, chloride and bicarbonate. Substances whose concentrations decrease with increased flow rate include phosphate and urea. Potassium concentration does not change with increased flow rate.

4. B

Coeliac disease is a T-cell mediated autoimmune disease of the small bowel where prolamine intolerance causes villous atrophy and malabsorption. Duodenal biopsy at endoscopy will show subtotal villous atrophy, increased intra-epithelial white blood cells and crypt hyperplasia which will reverse on a gluten-free diet.

5. D

This patient has gastro-oesophageal reflux disease. It is caused by multiple factors including loss of oesophageal peristaltic function, smoking and alcohol which leads to reflux of stomach contents. Helicobacter pylori infection is typically associated with peptic ulcers. Absence of oesophageal peristalsis is indicative of achalasia. Protrusion of the stomach into the thorax is associated with hiatus hernia and Barrett's oesophagus involves the replacement of mucosa with metaplastic columnar epithelium.

6. C

The abdominal aorta begins at T12 and ends at L4 bifurcating into left and right common iliac arteries. The coeliac artery is at the level of T12 and supplies the liver, spleen, superior pancreas and superior duodenum. The superior mesenteric artery arises at L1 and supplies the distal duodenum, jejuno-ileum, ascending colon and part of the transverse colon. The gonadal arteries are surprisingly situated high up in the abdomen at L2. The inferior mesenteric artery arises at L3 and supplies the large intestine.

7. D

Parietal cells are found in gastric glands that line the fundus and body of the stomach. These cells secrete intrinsic factor which is necessary for the absorption of vitamin B12 in the ileum.

EMQ

This question is based on the different types of secretions in the gastrointestinal tract.

8. J

The cephalic phase results from the detection and ingestion of food. This is stimulated via the vagus nerve to the stomach causing enterochromaffin-like cell to secrete acid and G cells to secrete gastrin.

9. F

Secretin regulates the pH of the duodenum by inhibiting secretion of gastric acid from parietal cells of the stomach and by stimulating production of bicarbonate from the pancreas.

10. B

Gastrin stimulates the parietal cells of the stomach to secrete acid and also indirectly by binding on to gastrin receptors on enterochromaffin-like cells in the stomach which causes release of histamine.

Cardiovascular System (Chapter 8)

1.
   a. Hydrostatic pressure forces water out of the capillaries whereas osmotic pressure drives water back into the vessels. (1) The balance between these two forces differs at different points on the capillaries and is created by the direction of blood flow and imbalance in solutes which favours the formation of interstitial fluid (1)
   b. One mark for each correct curve: total of two marks.

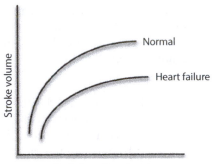

End-diastolic volume

   c. In heart failure the elevated venous pressure increases capillary hydrostatic pressure. (1) If the resulting extravasation of fluid is greater than the ability of the lymphatic system to return this fluid to the vascular space, oedema will result (1)
   d. Angiotensin II constricts the efferent arteriole causing a decrease in renal blood flow (RBF) and increase in glomerular filtration rate (GFR). ACE inhibitors inhibit formation of angiotensin II therefore dilating efferent arteriole resulting in a rise in RBF (1) and a decrease in GFR (1)
   e. Any one of the following examples with mechanism of action scores two marks:
   Loop diuretics – inhibits Na^+–K^+–$2CL^-$ cotransporter in thick ascending limb of the loop of Henle therefore inhibiting sodium, chloride and potassium reabsorption.
   Thiazide diuretic – inhibits reabsorption of sodium and chloride from distal convoluted tubule by acting on Na^+-Cl^- transporter.

This question focuses on heart failure, a condition where the heart fails to maintain an adequate circulation for the needs of the body despite an adequate filling pressure. There are many causes of failure, for example, hypertension, arrhythmias, but ischaemic heart disease is the primary cause of systolic heart failure. The pathophysiology of heart failure is complex, involving systolic or diastolic dysfunction and neuro-hormonal activation. The symptoms of this condition depend on whether it is left or right heart failure but it is rare for any part of the heart to fail in isolation.

2.
   a. Staphylococcus aureus (1)
   b. Blood cultures (1)
   c. Echocardiogram (1)
   d. Any one of the following scores half a mark: total of two marks.
      Murmur
      Fever
      Osler's nodes
      Roth's spots
      Janeway's lesions
      Clubbing
      Splinter or subungual haemorrhage
      Splenomegaly
   e. Any one of the following scores half a mark: total of two marks.
      Myocardial infarction
      Arrhythmias
      Congestive heart failure
      Pericarditis
      Glomerulonephritis
      Acute kidney injury
      Aortic root or myocardial abscesses
      Stroke
   f. Enterotoxin (1)
   g. Streptococcus pyogenes (1)
   h. Superantigen toxin allows the non-specific binding of MHC II with
      T-cell receptors resulting in polyclonal T-cell activation which causes a
      cytokine storm followed by a multisystem disease (1)

This question focuses on infective endocarditis. Any fever with a new murmur
is deemed as endocarditis until proven otherwise. Many bacteria can cause
endocarditis but streptococcus viridians is the most common cause. Other
bacteria include staphylococcus aureus/epidermidis, enterococcus. Diagnosis
is based on the Duke criteria which include all major and minor criteria.
Antibiotic prophylaxis to prevent infective endocarditis is not recommended
as there is no proven association between interventional procedures and
development of infective endocarditis.

3.
   a. Due to abnormalities in separation of the truncus arteriosus into the
      aorta and pulmonary arteries (1)
   b. Pulmonary stenosis (½)
      Ventricular septal defect (½)
      Right ventricular hypertrophy (½)
      Over-riding aorta (½)
   c. Due to de-oxygenated blood bypassing the lungs and entering the systemic
      circulation (1)

d.

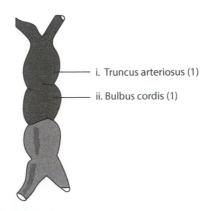

i. Truncus arteriosus (1)

ii. Bulbus cordis (1)

e. Caudocephalic folding brings the tube into the thoracic region (1)
   Lateral folding creates a heart tube (1)
f. Any one of the following scores one mark: total of two marks.
   Transposition of the great vessels
   Pulmonary valve atresia
   Tricuspid atresia
   Total anomalous pulmonary venous drainage
   Truncus arteriosus
   Hypoplastic left heart

This question focuses on congenital heart defects. These defects can be classified as either a left to right (acyanotic) or right to left (cyanotic) shunt. Left to right shunt requires a hole, and blood from the left heart is returned to the lungs instead of going to the body resulting in increased pulmonary artery or pulmonary venous pressure. Examples of this shunt include atrial septal defect, ventricular septal defect and patent ductus arteriosus. Right to left shunt requires a hole and a distal obstruction where de-oxygenated blood bypasses the lungs.

4.
   a. This increase in mass predominantly results from a chronic increase in afterload of the left ventricle caused by the hypertension (1)
   b. Left fifth intercostal space in midclavicular line (1)
   c. Displaced apex beat (1)
      S4 heart sound (1)
   d. Sympathetic nerve activation (1)
      Decreased renal perfusion pressure (1)
      Decreased sodium delivery to distal tubules of kidney (1)
   e. Renin activates the renin-angiotensin system by cleaving angiotensinogen to produce angiotensin I (1)
   f. Minoxidil (1)
      Hydralazine (1)

This question is based on hypertension. All patients with a blood pressure of ≥160/100 mmHg should be treated. For patients who have ≥140/90 mmHg, the decision to treat is based on the risk of coronary events, the presence of diabetes or end-organ damage. Isolated systolic hypertension is the most common form of hypertension and is due to the atherosclerosis. Around 95% of cases have an unknown cause but secondary hypertension (~5%) can be due to renal or endocrine diseases. There are various treatments available including calcium channel blockers, ACE inhibitors and diuretics with the goal of aiming for a blood pressure of <140/90 mmHg or <130/80 mmHg in diabetics.

5.
    a. ECG (1)
    b. Any one of the following scores one mark:
    ST depression
    Flat or inverted T waves
    c. Nitric oxide (1) causing venodilation (1)
    d. Ejection systolic murmur (1)
    Aortic valve closes when the aortic pressure is greater than the left ventricular pressure (1)
    e. Second (1)
    f. i. Fifth intercostal space left midclavicular line (1)
    ii. Second intercostal space left sternal border (1)
    g. NICE provides guidance on whether the drug can be recommended to be provided by hospitals based on cost-effectiveness and clinical evidence (1)

This question focuses on angina which presents as central tightness or heaviness that is brought on by exertion or relieved by rest. Angina can be classified as either stable (angina that is brought on by effort and relieved by rest), unstable (angina that occurs with minimal exertion or at rest), decubitus (angina that is precipitated by lying flat) or prinzmetal (caused by coronary artery spasm). Investigations usually include ECG initially, however patients that present with atypical pain may undergo exercise testing or functional imaging, for example, a stress echocardiogram.

6.
    a. Left femoral vein, left external iliac vein, left common iliac vein, inferior vena cava, right atrium, right ventricle, pulmonary artery (2)
    b. Ratio of air ventilation to local blood flow in a respiratory area of the lungs (1)
    In pulmonary embolism, ventilation rate is normal but blood flow is decreased to area supplied by artery which has been partially/completely occluded by embolism (1)
    c. Sinus tachycardia (1)
    d. Respiratory alkalosis (1) due to hyperventilation causing lowered arterial pCO_2 (1)
    e. Warfarin inhibits hepatic synthesis of vitamin K-dependent clotting factors II, VII. IX and X by inhibiting vitamin K epoxide reductase (1)
    Aim for INR 2–3 (1)
    Continue for at least six weeks (1)

This question focuses on DVT which may present with calf warmth/tenderness/swelling/erythema and pitting oedema. The risk of a DVT can be calculated using the Wells score where ≤1 point indicates an unlikely DVT but ≥2 points indicates a likely DVT. In addition, a D-dimer measurement is a sensitive but not specific test which when combined with Well's score is sufficient to exclude a DVT. Treatment is typically with LMWH combined with warfarin where LMWH is stopped once INR is 2–3. A below-knee DVT is typically treated for at least six weeks whereas an above-knee DVT is treated for at least three months.

7.
   a. This is due to atherosclerosis causing stenosis of arteries therefore reduced blood supply to muscle (1)
   b. Intermittent claudication (1)
   c. Any one of the following scores half a mark: total of one mark.
      Hypertension
      High cholesterol
      Obesity
      Family history of peripheral artery disease, stroke or heart disease
   d. Colour duplex ultrasound scan (1)
   e. Dorsalis pedis (1) – lateral to extensor hallucis longus tendon (1)
      Posterior tibial (1) – posterior to medial malleolus (1)
      Popliteal (1) – deep palpation in midline within popliteal fossa (1)

This question focuses on peripheral arterial disease. Typically, patients complain of a cramping pain in the calf, thigh or buttock after walking for a certain distance. Calf pain that is relieved by rest suggests femoral disease while buttock claudication suggests iliac disease. Tests include basic bloods and an ankle-brachial pressure index. Management includes modifying risk factors, exercise programmes, vasoactive drugs and surgery.

8.
   a. Rate of injection of blood into the aorta is decreased as a result of a poorly functioning ventricle therefore duration of ejection is prolonged so amplitude of pulse is diminished (1)
   b. Chest pain (angina) results from the increased oxygen requirement due to hypertrophic myocardium (1)
      Syncope results when systemic vasodilation in the presence of a fixed stroke volume causes arterial systolic blood pressure to fall (1)
   c. Any one of the following scores half a mark: total of one mark.
      Senile calcification
      Bicuspid valve
      Rheumatic heart disease
   d. Ejection systolic murmur (1) – due to the turbulence that occurs as blood flows across the stenotic valve (1)
   e. Depolarisation of plasma membrane causes opening of plasma L-type calcium channels in T-tubules resulting in influx of calcium into cytosol. (1) Calcium binds to ryanodine receptors on the sarcoplasmic

reticulum causing opening of calcium channels intrinsic to these receptors (calcium-induced calcium release). (1) The influx of calcium into cytosol induces myocyte contraction (1)

   f. Sarco-endoplasmic reticulum calcium ATPase pump (1)

This question focuses on aortic stenosis which typically presents with syncope, angina and heart failure. Patients may show signs of a slow rising pulse with a narrow pulse pressure, a heaving non-displaced apex beat and an ejection systolic murmur that radiates to the carotids. When the aortic valve becomes stenotic, resistance to systolic ejection occurs and a systolic pressure gradient develops between the left ventricle and the aorta. This outflow obstruction leads to an increase in left ventricular systolic pressure.

9.
   a. Continuous ('machinery') murmur (1)
   b. PDA allows blood to go from the systemic circulation to the pulmonary circulation (left to right shunt). (1) The ductus arteriosus connects the pulmonary artery to the descending aorta therefore allowing blood from the right ventricle to bypass the lungs (1)
   c. Ductus venosus (1) – shunts a portion of the left umbilical vein blood flow directly to the inferior vena cava therefore allowing oxygenated blood from the placenta to bypass the liver (1)
     Foramen ovale (1) – allows blood to enter the left atrium from the right atrium (1)
   d. Left sixth aortic arch (1)
   e. Any one of the following scores one mark: total of two marks.
     Ventricular septal defect
     Atrial septal defect
     Atrioventricular defect

This question focuses on patent ductus arteriosus, a congenital heart defect. This is an example of a left to right shunt defect which is characterised by a leak of blood from the systemic circulation into the pulmonary circulation. This results in an increased blood volume and pressure within the pulmonary circulation resulting in pulmonary hypertension. The ductus arteriosus is a normal structure in foetal life that closes by 2–3 weeks after birth.

10.
   a. Group A beta-haemolytic streptococci (1)
   b. Rheumatic fever causing damage to valves resulting in thickening and fibrosis leading to stenosis or regurgitation. The resultant valvular heart disease leads to heart failure (1)
   c. Systolic dysfunction is causing decreased ejection fraction, hence increased volume of blood in the left ventricle which backs up to the left atrium and pulmonary veins. (1) The resulting hydrostatic pressure favours extravasation of fluid into lung parenchyma causing pulmonary oedema which impairs gas exchange (1)
   d. Atrial fibrillation (1) – absent P waves (1)

   e. Sternocleidomastoid muscle (1)
      Elevated JVP is a sign of venous hypertension (right sided failure) (1)
   f. Any one of the following scores one mark: total of two marks.
      To reduce mortality rates
      To reduce concordance with treatment or medical advice
      To reduce use of medical and nursing services
      To reduce stress or distress
      To reduce risk of developing mental health problems

This question focuses on rheumatic fever. Pharyngeal infection with group A beta-haemolytic streptococci triggers rheumatic fever 2–4 weeks later. Diagnosis is based on Jones criteria where there are major and minor criteria. Management involves bed rest, antibiotics and analgesia. The most common complications include carditis, mitral stenosis and congestive heart failure.

MCQ

1. D

Bacterial endocarditis involving the tricuspid valve is likely due to illicit intravenous drug use. Staphylococcus aureus is responsible for most cases of endocarditis in intravenous drug users. Tricuspid valve endocarditis is uncommon in non-drug users but may occur in patients with pacemakers, central venous lines or haemodialysis.

2. B

Coarctation of the aorta is typically located in the thoracic aorta distal to the origin of the left subclavian artery. In early onset of coarctation of aorta a chest X-ray may show cardiomegaly and pulmonary oedema whereas in late onset rib notching secondary to collateral vessels is seen.

3. D

This scenario is classical of acute myocardial infarction (MI) with symptoms and signs of cardiogenic shock. In this case there is cardiovascular collapse associated with shock which is seen in patients with acute MI due to papillary muscle rupture. The ECG findings suggest an inferior MI where the majority are due to occlusion of the right coronary artery. However, it may be due to occlusion of the left circumflex artery (LCA) but the absence of a reciprocal ST depression in lead I would be more suggestive of a LCA occlusion.

4. A

Only Prinzmetal's angina causes ST elevation. All other options cause ST depression.

5. A

Brain natriuretic peptide (BNP) is an active peptide that has vasodilator and natriuretic properties. BNP can be raised in cardiac conditions such as heart failure, acute coronary syndromes and atrial fibrillation. It may be raised in non-cardiac conditions such as acute pulmonary embolism and sepsis. All statements are true except option A as it induces vasodilation.

6. D

Superior vena cava because blood is going to a more metabolically active area leading to increased oxygen extraction.

7. E

Transposition of the great arteries involves the transposition of the aorta and pulmonary artery so that the aorta arises from the right ventricle and the pulmonary artery arises from the left ventricle. All options are possible treatment options. Prostaglandin E keeps the connection between the aorta and pulmonary open therefore allowing intracardiac mixing.

EMQ

This question is based on valvular heart disease.

8. G

This scenario describes carcinoid syndrome which occurs secondary to carcinoid tumours. Patients may experience cardiac abnormalities due to serotonin-induced fibrosis, which is filtered by the lungs and rarely reaches the left side heart valves. This syndrome typically causes tricuspid insufficiency and pulmonary stenosis.

9. A

Aortic stenosis presents with classic triad of syncope, angina and dyspnoea. On examination patients show an ejection systolic murmur (i.e. crescendo–decrescendo) best heard at the right second intercostal space radiating to the carotids. The second heart sound is generated by the closing of the aortic valve therefore a stenotic valve may cause the second heart sound to become quieter. Other causes of systolic murmurs include pulmonary stenosis, mitral valve prolapse and tricuspid regurgitation.

10. D

This scenario describes mitral regurgitation, which is typically associated with ischaemic heart disease and a dilated left ventricle. Patients present with peripheral oedema, flushed face and an irregularly irregular pulse consistent with atrial fibrillation. The apex beat is usually displaced and thrusting in nature. On auscultation there will be a holosystolic murmur loudest at the apex radiating to the axilla.

Respiratory System (Chapter 9)

1.
   a. One mark for correct axis
      one mark for each correct curve.

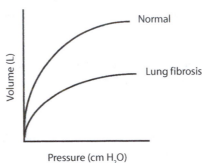

   b. i. Decreased (1)
      ii. Decreased (1)
   c. Low compliance (high elastic recoil) (1)
   d. Decreased capacity of lung to transfer gas across alveoli (1)
   e. Alveolar epithelium (1)
      Interstitial space (1)
      Capillary endothelium (1)

This question focuses on the lung mechanics. At the resting expiratory level three forces are in equilibrium: (1) lungs pull in and up, (2) thoracic cage pulls out and (3) diaphragm pulls down. Inspiration is an active process as a result of the contraction of the diaphragm and intercostal muscles whereas expiration is a passive process. Lung compliance is defined as the stretchiness of the lungs and a high compliance indicates a pliable lung (low elastic recoil) whereas low compliance indicates a stiff lung (high elastic recoil).

2.
   a. Damage to recurrent laryngeal nerve (1)
   b. Lymphatic supply to the area (1)
      Blood supply to the area (1)
      Access to coelomic space (1)
   c. Bronchial airway obstruction by tumour (1)
   d. TNM is a cancer staging system (½)
      Tis – Tumour in situ; N0 – No lymph node involvement; M0 – No metastatis (½)
   e. Squamous cell – 35% (1)
      Adenocarcinoma – 27% (1)
      Small cell – 20% (1)
      Large cell – 10% (1)

This question focuses on lung tumours which account for ~19% of all cancers. Cigarette smoking is the major risk factor. Types of lung tumours include squamous, adenocarcinoma, small cell, large cell and alveolar cell carcinoma. Many complications can occur as a consequence of a lung tumour such as recurrent laryngeal nerve palsy, phrenic nerve palsy, SVC obstruction and Horner's syndrome (Pancoast tumour). Prognosis is particularly worse with small cell carcinoma with a median survival of three months if untreated.

3.
   a. Tobacco smoking (1)
   b. Any one of the following scores one mark: total of two marks.
      Epithelial thickening
      Mucous gland hypertrophy
      Prominence of airway smooth musculature
      Fibrosis of bronchioles
   c. Type 2 respiratory failure (1)
   d. Compensated respiratory acidosis (1)
      In response to a respiratory acidosis due to carbon dioxide retention secondary to COPD, the kidneys will start to retain more bicarbonate in order to correct the pH (1)
   e. Central chemoreceptors – medulla oblongata (1)
      Peripheral chemoreceptors – carotid bodies and aortic arch (1)
   f. The central chemoreceptors adapt to a persistent increased carbon dioxide level (1) and now the main drive for respiration changes to low PO_2 acting on peripheral chemoreceptors (1)

This question focuses on COPD, a condition that comprises chronic bronchitis and emphysema. Chronic bronchitis is defined as productive cough on most days for 3 months of 2 successive years. Emphysema is defined as enlarged air spaces distal to terminal bronchioles with destruction of alveolar walls. COPD can be classified as either pink puffers or blue bloaters. Pink puffers have increased alveolar ventilation, a normal PO_2 and a normal or low PCO_2. Blue bloaters have decreased alveolar ventilation, a low PO_2 and a high PCO_2.

4.
   a. Cyanosis (1)
   b. Asthma results from airway obstruction due to bronchospasms that results in increased mucus secretion and oedema of the respiratory mucosa. (1) The build-up of mucus in the alveoli creates a V/Q mismatch leading to hypoxia when the body's response is to increase heart rate to increase ventilation (1)
   c. Any one of the following scores half a mark: total of two marks.
      Anaemia
      Acute respiratory distress disorder
      Pneumothorax
      Pulmonary embolism
      Pulmonary oedema
   d. Bronchi (½) and bronchioles (½)
   e. Any one of the following score half a mark: total of two marks.

    Goblet cell hyperplasia
    Hypertrophy of submucosal glands and smooth muscle
    Mucus plugs
    Squamous metaplasia
    Thickened basement membrane

f. Corticosteroids – decrease number of cytokines and macrophages therefore reducing inflammation (1)

    B2 adrenoceptor agonists – increase sympathetic stimulation causing bronchodilation (1)

This question focuses on asthma, a condition caused by reversible airways obstruction. The pathophysiology involves bronchial muscle contraction, mucosal swelling/inflammation and increased mucus production. In acute settings, asthma is classified as severe attack, life-threatening or near fatal and these are based on various signs such as respiratory rate, heart rate and peak expiratory flow measurement. Chronic management of asthma is based on a stepwise approach set by the British Thoracic society.

5.

    a. Any one of the following scores half a mark: total of one mark.
       Pneumonia
       Tuberculosis
       Pulmonary infarction
       Rheumatoid arthritis
       Bronchogenic carcinoma
       Lymphoma

    b. Visceral – vagus nerve and sympathetic trunk (1)
       Parietal – intercostal and phrenic nerves (1)

    c. The seventh to the ninth intercostal space superior to the rib in the midaxillary line (1) to avoid the neurovascular bundle that runs along the inferior margin (1)

    d. Skin → fat → External intercostal muscle → internal intercostal muscle →endothoracic fascia → parietal pleura (2)

    e. Referred pain which spreads to the dermatome of the umbilical region as they are supplied by the same segment of the spinal cord (1)

    f. Phrenic nerve (1) from cervical nerves C3, C4, C5 (1)

This question focuses on pleural effusion, which is classified as either transudate or exudate. Causes of transudates include cardiac failure, fluid overload, cirrhosis and nephrotic syndrome. Exudates are due to increased leakiness of pleural capillaries secondary to malignancy, inflammation or infection. On examination there will be decreased expansion, stony dull percussion and reduced breath sounds. All pleural fluid aspirated should be sent for clinical chemistry, bacteriology and cytology.

6.

    a. Any correct answers scores half a mark: total of two marks.
       A – Pseudostratified ciliated columnar epithelium

      B – Mucous glands in the submucosa
      C – Hyaline cartilage
      D – Smooth muscle

  b. Inhalation of asbestos fibres causes chronic inflammation leading to fibrosis (1)

  c. Any of three of the following scores one mark:
      Viridans streptococci
      Neisseria
      Moraxella
      Corynebacteria
      Anaerobes
      Candida albicans
      Streptococcus pneumoniae
      Streptococcus pyogenes
      Haemophilus influenzae

  d. PaO_2 will decrease and $PaCO_2$ will increase, resulting in respiratory acidosis (1)

  e. At lower pH, O_2 dissociates more readily from haemoglobin whereas in an alkaline environment association of oxygen with haemoglobin is favoured (1)

  f. Restrictive (1)
      Reduced forced vital capacity (FVC) and reduced forced expiratory volume at the end of the first second (FEV_1) (1)

  g. Any one of the following scores one mark: total of two marks.
      Stigma
      Demands of coping with physical aspects and treatments
      Psychological aspects such as anxiety and depression, impact on identity
      Impact on relationships (i.e. sufferers become increasingly reliant on family but relationships also become increasingly strained)
      Change of roles within the family

This question focuses on an important concept, the oxygen-haemoglobin dissociation curve. This curve demonstrates the saturation percentage of haemoglobin at various partial pressures of oxygen. At high partial pressures of oxygen, haemoglobin binds to oxygen forming oxyhaemoglobin. The partial pressure of oxygen drops as red blood cells travel to tissues in demand of oxygen, hence the oxyhaemoglobin releases oxygen. Many factors influence oxygen binding and it is important to note factors that cause a left and right shift of the curve, for example, decreased temperature and decreased pH cause a left shift whereas an increased temperature and increased pH cause a right shift.

7.
  a. Alveolar macrophages (1)
      Nasal mucosa (1)
      Mucociliary epithelium lining (goblet cells, submucosal seromucous glands) (1)

  b. Any one of the following scores one mark: total of two marks.
     Reduced chest expansion
     Dull percussion note
     Increased tactile vocal fremitus/vocal resonance
     Bronchial breathing
  c. All three correct for one mark.
     Streptococcus pneumoniae
     Haemophilus influenzae
     Mycoplasma pneumoniae
  d. Inhibition of bacterial cell wall synthesis (1)
  e. Any one of the below scores one mark: total of three marks.
     Complexity of medication regimen
     Lack of immediate benefit of therapy
     Experienced/perceived side effects
     Fear of dependence
     Any physical factors limiting administration, for example, visual
     impairment

This question focuses on pneumonia which is a lower respiratory tract
illness. Pneumonia can be classified as either community acquired or hospital
acquired. Common organisms that cause community acquired pneumonia
include streptococcus pneumoniae, haemophilus influenzae, mycoplasma
pneumoniae and staphylococcus aureus. Hospital acquired pneumonia is
commonly caused by gram-negative enterobacteria or staphylococcus aureus
but may include pseudomonas and klebsiella. CURB-65 is a simple scoring
system to assess the severity of the illness. A score of 2 or more would usually
require hospital admission.

  8.
    a. Tension pneumothorax. (1) There are signs of respiratory distress and
       tracheal deviation with associated trauma (1)
    b. Peripheral – diminished blood flow to a local area causing bluish discol-
       oration only to extremities or fingers (1)
       Central – diminished arterial oxygen saturation leading to bluish discol-
       oration around lips and tongue (1)
    c. Insert a large-bore needle into the second intercostal space in the mid-
       clavicular line on the left side of the chest (1)
    d. Tracheal deviation is an indicator of upper mediastinal shift. (1)
       Mediastinum pushed over to contralateral hemithorax compressing
       great veins leading to cardiorespiratory arrest (1)
    e. Synchondrosis (1)
    f. Sternocleidomastoid (½), scalene (½), pectoralis major (½), pectoralis
       minor (½)

This question focuses on tension pneumothorax, which is a medical emergency
that requires immediate treatment. This occurs in situations such as patients
who are ventilated, trauma patients, blocked or displaced chest drains and

patients with underlying lung disease. Patients present with severe symptoms and signs of respiratory distress and management should not be delayed by obtaining a chest X-ray. Immediate management is insertion of a large-bore needle into the second intercostal space in the midclavicular line on the side of the suspected pneumothorax. A chest drain is then inserted usually at the fifth intercostal space in the midaxillary line. This aims to help restore haemodynamic and respiratory stability by optimising ventilation/perfusion and minimising mediastinal shift.

9.
  a. Right lower lobe consolidation (1)
  b. Any one of the following scores one mark: total of two marks.
     Bronchial breathing
     Decreased air entry
     Crepitations

  c. $7.25 = 6.1 + \log\left(\dfrac{[HCO_3^-]}{0.03 \times 66}\right)$

     $(7.25 - 6.1) + 0.297 = \log [HCO_3^-]$ (1)
     $[HCO_3^-] = 10^{1.447} = 27.99$ mmol/L (1)
     Acid-base balance – partially compensated respiratory acidosis (1)
  d. Streptococcus pneumoniae (1)
  e. Amoxicillin (1)
  f. Macrolide (1) – inhibits protein synthesis (1)

This question focuses on pneumonia. Clinical features of this condition include fever, rigors, malaise, dyspnoea, cough, purulent sputum, haemoptysis and pleuritic pain. On examination there may be pyrexia, tachypnoea, tachycardia, hypotension and signs of consolidation. Pneumonia is treated with antibiotics, typically amoxicillin if mild. However, if severity increases this may include the addition of clarithromycin or doxycycline or if severe will require intravenous antibiotics such as co-amoxiclav.

10.

  a. Pseudostratified ciliated columnar (1)
  b. Malignant (1)
  c. Left recurrent laryngeal nerve damage causes hoarseness (1)
     Phrenic nerve damage causes shortness of breath (1)
  d. FEV_1:FVC ratio more than 70% (1) indicating a restrictive
     lung disease (1)
  e. Spirometry (1)
     Peak flow meter (1)
  f. Oblique fissure – T3 vertebrae to sixth costochondral junction (1)
     Horizontal fissure – from oblique fissure in midaxillary line to fourth
     costal cartilage (1)

This question focuses on an important point in the surface markings of the lung. The pleura starts above the mid-point of the medial third of the clavicle and meets in the midline at the second rib. The left side then diverges at rib four while the right continues to the sixth rib. Both left and right cross the eighth rib at the midclavicular line, the tenth rib in the midaxillary line and reach the posterior chest just below the twelfth rib. The surface marking of the lungs is two rib spaces less than the pleura. The oblique fissure separates the inferior lobe of the lung from the superior and middle lobe whereas the horizontal fissure separates the superior from the middle lobe.

MCQ

1. C

The thoracic duct enters the thorax through the aortic hiatus of the diaphragm in the posterior mediastinum. As it ascends through the thorax it enters the superior mediastinum. The superior mediastinum contains neural, vascular and respiratory structures such as the thymus, trachea and thoracic duct. The anterior mediastinum contains no major structures. The middle mediastinum contains several important organs, vessels, nerves and lymphatic structures such as the heart, pericardium, ascending aorta, pulmonary trunk and superior vena cava. The posterior mediastinum contains the thoracic aorta, oesophagus, azygos system of veins and sympathetic trunk.

2. A

The right main bronchus is wider and more vertical than the left hence foreign objects are more likely to be aspirated into the right main bronchus. The superior segmental bronchus of the lower lobar bronchus exits from the posterior wall of the lobar bronchi hence foreign objects are most likely to enter this segment if aspiration occurs when patients are in a supine position.

3. E

The functional residual capacity is the volume of air in the lungs at the end of expiration. This volume cannot be expired entirely hence cannot be measured by spirometry. However, this can be measured by the helium dilution technique.

4. B

The waveforms of jugular venous pressure consist of the *a*, *c* and *v* waves and *x* and *y* descents. The A wave represents presystolic (produced by right atrial contraction), the *c* wave represents bulging of the tricuspid valve into the right atrium during ventricular systole and the *v* wave occurs in late systole. The *x* descent represents the start of atrial relaxation during ventricular systole. The *y* descent occurs when the tricuspid valve opens and blood flows into the right ventricle. In pulmonary hypertension you would expect to see large *a* waves.

Absence of *a* waves occurs in atrial fibrillation, slow *y* descent occurs in tricuspid stenosis and right atrial myxoma, and prominent *v* waves occur in tricuspid regurgitation.

5. E

Emphysema is a cause of obstructive lung disease. Typically, a reduction in FEV_1 hence a decreased FEV_1:FVC ratio will be seen. In addition the residual volume is increased. The destruction of the alveolar capillary bed will show a reduced diffuse capacity of the lung for carbon monoxide (DLCO).

6. C

This scenario describes pneumonia. Signs that are associated with this condition are pyrexia, cyanosis confusion, tachypnoea, tachycardia, hypotension and signs of consolidation (dull percussion note, increased tactile vocal fremitus/vocal resonance, bronchial breathing, diminished chest expansion).

7. B

Cystic fibrosis is an autosomal recessive condition caused by mutations in the cystic fibrosis transmembrane ductance regulator (CFTR) gene on chromosome 7. CFTR is a chloride channel with a defect leading to defective chloride secretion and increased sodium absorption across airway epithelium. Many complications occur such as recurrent infections, bronchiectasis, pancreatic insufficiency and male infertility. It is estimated that today patients live into their mid-40s or 50s.

EMQ

This question is based on the various examples of lung conditions.

8. E

This scenario describes pleural effusion. On examination there will be decreased expansion, stony dull percussion and diminished breath sounds on the affected side. With large effusions there may be tracheal deviation away from the effusion. Chest X-ray will show blunting of costophrenic angles.

9. C

This scenario describes tension pneumothorax. On examination, a pneumothorax will show reduced expansion, hyper-resonance and diminished breath sounds on the affected side. With a tension pneumothorax the trachea will be deviated away from the affected side and the patient will be very unwell.

10. I

This scenario describes bronchiectasis. Patients will present with a persistent cough with purulent sputum and intermittent haemoptysis. On examination you may notice finger clubbing, coarse inspiratory crepitations and wheeze.

Urology (Chapter 10)

1.
   a. Correct labelling of glomerulus scores one mark

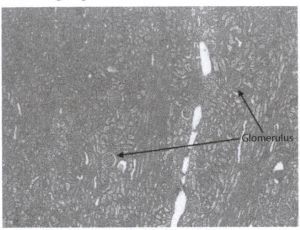

   b. Podocytes (1)
   c. Type 2 – Goodpasture's syndrome (1)
      Type 3 – Membranous glomerulonephritis or poststreptococcal glomer-
      ulonephritis (1)
   d. Glomerular capillary endothelial cells (1)
      Glomerular basement membrane (1)
      Podocytes (1)
   e. Large in size (1)
      Negatively charged (1)
   f. Increased urine output and osmolality (1)

This question focuses on the glomerulus structure. Blood plasma enters the
afferent arteriole and flows into the glomerulus. The Bowman's capsule consists of a visceral and parietal layer that surround the glomerulus. The visceral
layer is made up of podocytes that form slits allowing fluid to pass through
into the nephron. This fluid then leaves the glomerulus through the efferent
arteriole.

2.
   a. Metabolic acidosis (1)
   b. $140 + 6.5 - (99 + 16.5) = 31$ mmol/L (1)
   c. Any one of the following scores one mark: total of two marks.
      Lactic acid (shock, infection, tissue ischaemia)
      Renal failure
      Diabetes mellitus
      Drugs/toxins (salicylates, methanol)
   d. Labelling of each correct pump scores one mark: total of three marks.

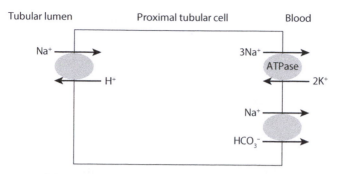

Tubular lumen — Proximal tubular cell — Blood

e. Any one of the following scores one mark:
   Oliguric renal failure
   K⁺ sparing diuretics
   Rhabdomyolysis
   Addison's disease
   Burns
   Drugs, for example, ACE inhibitor
   Insulin (1) – Reduces K+ by activating Na⁺/K⁺-ATPase pumps resulting in cellular uptake of potassium (1)

This question focuses on acid-base balance. A simple method to determine the acid-base balance is based on looking at the pH (<7.35 = acidosis, >7.45 = alkalosis), then looking at the CO_2 (if there is an abnormality that is consistent for the pH this is likely a respiratory cause) and finally looking at the HCO_3 (if there is an abnormality that is consistent with the pH this is likely a metabolic cause). The anion gap is calculated as the difference between the cations and anions and is useful in determining the cause of a metabolic acidosis.

3.
   a. Kidney (1)
   b. The ureter begins its descent to the bladder by running along the medial aspect of the psoas muscle. (1) Here the ureter lies anteriorly and slightly medial to the tips of the L2–L5 transverse processes. (1) It enters the pelvis anteriorly to the sacroiliac joint at the bifurcation of the common iliac vessels (at the pelvic brim) and then courses anteriorly to the internal iliac artery down lateral pelvic sidewall (1)
   c. Decrease in glomerular filtration rate (GFR) (1) – obstruction causes increase in intraluminal ureteral pressure. This increased pressure is transmitted directly to nephron tubules. As pressure in the proximal tubule and Bowman space increase, GFR falls (1)
   d. Regulation at distal convoluted tubule (1)
      Transporters – Plasma membrane Ca^{2+} ATPase (PMCA), sodium-calcium exchanger (NCX) (1)
   e. Parathyroid hormone from parathyroid gland (1)
      Calcitonin from parafollicular cells of thyroid gland (1)

This question focuses on kidney stones. There are three main areas where stones deposit; (1) pelviureteric junction, (2) pelvic brim and (3) vesicoureteric junction. The most common types of stones include calcium oxalate, struvite, urate and hydroxyapatite. Patients typically present with renal colic, nausea and vomiting, haematuria and possibly a co-existing urinary tract infection. On examination there may be renal angle tenderness.

4.
  a. Blockage of renal arteries causes the kidney to increase production of renin (1) which causes a cascade of events leading to peripheral vasoconstriction and fluid retention causing an increase in blood pressure (1)
  b. Renin is a hormone (1) that converts angiotensinogen to angiotensin I (1)
  c. Angiotensin II stimulates release of aldosterone from the adrenal cortex (1) Aldosterone causes the tubules of kidneys to reabsorb sodium and water into the blood and cause potassium secretion causing hypokalaemia (1)
  d. Stenotic lesions will lead to velocity increase (1) and post-stenotic turbulence (1)
  e. In renal artery stenosis the afferent pressure is reduced therefore autoregulation is dependent on changes in efferent arteriolar tone. (1) ACE inhibitors prevent formation of angiotensin II, which primarily causes vasoconstriction of efferent arterioles, therefore autoregulation is impaired, glomerular perfusion falls, renal ischaemic nephropathy develops and renal failure ensues (1)

This question focuses on renal artery stenosis, a condition that is largely caused by atherosclerosis. Patients may present with increased blood pressure resistant to treatment and worsening renal function after ACE inhibitor or angiotensin receptor blockers in bilateral renal artery stenosis. Other signs that may be present include flash pulmonary oedema, abdominal, carotid or femoral bruits.

5.
  a. Labelling of each correct element scores half a mark: total of two marks.

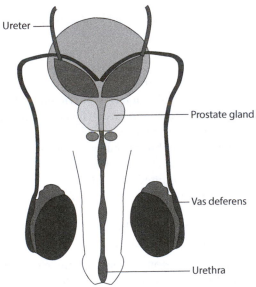

   b. Spongy, membranous, prostatic (1)
   c. Anterior – pubic symphysis (1)
      Posterior – wall of rectum (1)
      Superior – bladder (1)
   d. During the storage phase of micturition, sympathetic stimulation
      (hypogastric nerves) causes the internal urethral sphincter to contract
      and the detrusor muscle to relax. (1) During voiding phase, parasympa-
      thetic stimulation (pelvic nerves) causes the internal urethral sphincter
      to relax and the detrusor muscle to contract. (1) The pudendal nerve
      (S2–S4) (1) innervates the external urethral sphincter which relaxes
      under voluntary/somatic control to allow expulsion of urine (1)

This question focuses on micturition, a process that involves bladder filling and
initiation of a nervous reflex. The sympathetic postganglionic neurons release
noradrenaline that activate beta-3 adrenergic receptors causing bladder smooth
muscle. In addition, it also activates alpha-1 adrenergic receptors causing contraction of uretheral smooth muscle. Parasympathetic postganglionic neurons
release acetylcholine which stimulates M3 muscarinic receptors causing bladder
contraction. Somatic axons in the pudendal nerve release acetylcholine activating
nicotinic cholinergic receptors causing contraction of external sphincter muscle.

   6.
   a. Creatinine clearance – 19.40 ml/min (1)
      An eGFR of 45 indicates stage 3 chronic kidney disease (1)
   b. It increases urine osmolarity (1)
   c. Water will diffuse out from the cell and the cell will dehydrate and
      shrink (1)
   d. Antidiuretic hormone (1)
   e. Aquaporin-2 (1) acting on distal convoluted tubule and collecting
      ducts (1)
   f. i. C (1)
       ii. D (1)
       iii. I (1)

This question focuses on osmolality. The hypothalamic osmoreceptors senses
the plasma osmolality. In response either antidiuretic hormone (ADH) is
released or the thirst mechanism is activated acting on the kidney and brain
respectively. ADH will affect the renal water excretion whereas thirst will
affect water intake. ADH acts on the kidney to regulate the volume and osmolarity of the urine. If plasma ADH is low there will be large volume of urine
and if plasma ADH is high, small volume of urine is excreted. ADH increases
the permeability of the collecting duct and late distal tubule to water.

   7.
   a. Suprapubic catheterisation (1) through the abdominal wall (1)
   b. Any one of the following scores one mark: total of two marks.
      Enlarged, firm non-tender prostate on digital rectal examination
      Tender, warm prostate on digital rectal examination

Enlarged, nodular prostate on digital rectal examination
Oedema of penis with non-retractable foreskin
c. Prostate-specific antigen (1)
d. Sympathetic stimulation (hypogastric nerves) from T10–T12 causes the internal urethral sphincter to contract and the detrusor muscle to relax. (1) Parasympathetic stimulation (pelvic nerves) from S2–S4 causes the internal urethral sphincter to relax and the detrusor muscle to contract. (1)
The pudendal nerve (S2–S4) innervates the external urethral sphincter which relaxes under voluntary/somatic control to allow expulsion of urine (1)
e. Correct labelling of peripheral zone (1)

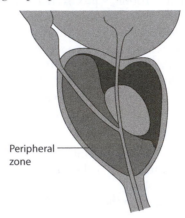

Peripheral zone

Early prostate cancer begins in the peripheral zone of the prostate so it does not cause urinary symptoms until it is more advance compared to benign prostatic hypertrophy which is more in the central zone so causes symptoms earlier (1)

This question focuses on urinary retention which is divided into either acute or chronic. Acute urinary retention is defined as painful inability to pass urine. There are many causes including prostatic enlargement, bladder or urethral stone impaction, urinary tract infection and pharmacological drugs such as anticholinergics. Chronic urinary retention is usually caused by bladder outlet obstruction, which can lead to hydronephrosis and renal impairment.

8.
a. Any one of the following scores half a mark: total of one mark.
Red blood cells
White blood cells
Crystals
Bacteria
Casts
b. Post-renal acute kidney injury (1)
c. 0.5ml–1ml/kg/hr (1)

d. The dramatic increase in urine output after the release of urinary tract obstruction (1), that is, post-obstructive diuresis
e. Ultrasound has no X-ray exposure whereas intravenous pyelogram involves the injection of contrast with subsequent X-rays taken (1)
f. Pelviureteric junction (1)
   Pelvic brim (1)
   Vesicoureteric junction (1)
g. A non-steroidal anti-inflammatory drug, for example, diclofenac, (1) inhibits enzyme cyclo-oxygenase thereby inhibiting formation of prostaglandins (1)

This question focuses on kidney stones. This is routinely diagnosed by CT scan which has largely replaced the intravenous urogram. The large majority of stones are visible on X-ray of the kidneys, ureters and bladder. There are two types of post-obstructive diuresis – physiological and pathological. Physiological diuresis is a response to solute and water overload whereas pathological diuresis is inappropriate diuresis of water beyond the euvolemic state.

9.
   a. Ureters run retroperitoneally (½)
      Pass inferiorly and lie on psoas (½)
      Relationship with testicular arteries, that is, ureter runs under the testicular vessels (½)
      Passes over bifurcation of common iliac artery (½)
   b. Any one of the following scores one mark: total of two marks.
      Citric acid: used by sperm for ATP production via the Krebs cycle
      Proteolytic enzymes (e.g. pepsinogen, lysozyme, amylase, hyaluronidase): to break down the clotting proteins from the seminal vesicles.
      Acid phosphatase: exact function is unknown.
   c. Wolffian duct → structures in males (any of the following): epididymis, vas deferens, ejaculatory duct and seminal vesicle (½)
      Müllerian duct → structures in females (any of the following): fallopian tubes, uterus and vagina (½)
   d. Gleason grading (1)
   e. Any of the following scores half a mark: total of one mark.
      Tubule formation
      Cell mitosis
      Nuclear pleomorphism
   f. Bone metastasis causing back pain (1)
      Prostatic venous plexus anastomoses with vertebral veins. (1) The veins lack valves (valveless veins of Batson) allowing backflow of blood (1)

MCQ

1. A

The membranous urethra is the least distensible portion of the urethra. This is due to the fact that the external sphincter surrounds it.

2. C

Highly reflective structures on ultrasound are termed hyperechoic whereas less reflective are termed hypoechoic. Examples of masses that are hypoechoic include renal adenomas, renal lymphomas and renal cysts. Renal cell carcinomas may be hyper- or hypoechogenic but the tumour pseudocapsule can sometimes be visualised as a hypoechoic halo. Renal angiomyolipoma are hypervascular lesions that tend to appear as hyperechoic lesions.

3. E

Obstructive hydronephrosis affects all aspects of renal function except urinary diluting ability. In addition, the glomerular filtration rate and renal blood flow are reduced.

4. D

There are five sites that renal stones are likely to lodge along the ureter. First the stones may impact in the calyx of the kidney followed by the ureteropelvic junction, pelvic brim, ureterovesicular junction and finally the vesical orifice.

5. B

The parathyroid hormone's (PTH) overall effect is to increase calcium and decrease phosphate, which is triggered by decreased serum ionised calcium. Actions of PTH include increasing osteoclast activity thereby releasing calcium and phosphate from bones, increasing calcium and decreasing phosphate reabsorption in the kidneys and increasing renal production of 1,25-dihydroxyvitamin D_3 (active metabolite of vitamin D).

6. C

Sympathetic postganglionic neurons release noradrenaline activating β -3 adrenergic receptors, which relax bladder smooth muscle. In addition, noradrenaline activates α-1 adrenergic receptors, which contract urethral smooth muscle. Parasympathetic postganglionic neurons release acetylcholine stimulating M3 muscarinic receptors in the bladder smooth muscle causing bladder contraction. Somatic axons in the pudendal nerve release acetylcholine activating nicotinic cholinergic receptors causing contraction of external sphincter muscle.

7. C

Decreased renal perfusion due to renal artery stenosis enhances angiotensin II production in which vaso constricts the efferent arterioles. This reduces renal blood flow but maintains glomerular filtration therefore the filtration rate is increased.

EMQ

This question is based on acid-base balance.

8. E

The pH indicates that this is acidosis. Whenever the PCO_2 and HCO_3 are abnormal in opposite directions then a mixed respiratory and metabolic acid-base disorder exists. In this case the PCO_2 is increased and HCO_3 is reduced hence a respiratory and metabolic acidosis coexist.

9. J

The pH indicates that this is alkalosis. The HCO_3 is above normal range indicating this is a metabolic alkalosis. Alkalaemia is sensed by central and peripheral chemoreceptors resulting in reduction in ventilation rate and therefore a rise in PCO_2 hence in this case there is associated respiratory compensation.

10. A

The pH indicates that this is acidosis. There is hypoxia and a rise in PCO_2 indicating this is respiratory acidosis.

Musculoskeletal System (Chapter 11)

1.
   a. Radial artery (½)
      Median nerve (½)
      Flexor carpi radialis tendon (½)
      Palmaris longus tendon (½)
   b. The palmar branch of the medican nerve is affected, which travels superficial to the flexor retinaculum of the hand (1)
   c. Flexor digitorum profundus (1)
      Flexor digitorum superficialis (1)
   d. Ulnar nerve unaffected (1)
   e. Thenar muscles (1)
      Lateral lumbricals (1)
   f. Within the hand there are excellent anastomoses between radial and ulnar arteries. (1) Anastomoses include superficial palmar arch, deep palmar arch, anterior and posterior carpal arches and posterior carpal arches (1)

This question focuses on the anatomy of the hand. The ulnar and radial arteries anastomose in the wrist to form arches. These arches combined with other branches to supply the hand and digits. The three main nerves that supply the hand include the ulnar, median and radial. The effect of cutting the ulnar nerve at the wrist involves motor loss, which includes the intrinsic muscles, except for those that supply the median nerve, which results in a claw hand. Sensory loss will be present on the medial side of the palm, palmar surface of the little and medial half of the ring fingers and the dorsal aspect of the distal and middle phalanges of these fingers. If the median is affected at the wrist there will be motor loss of the thenar muscles and the first and second lumbricals, which will result in wasting of the thenar muscles and inability to oppose the thumb. Sensory loss will be present on the lateral 3½ digits including their nail beds and the thenar area. If the radial nerve is affected at the wrist there will be no motor deficit, but only sensory loss will be present on the radial half of the dorsum of hand and dorsal aspect of radial 3½ digits.

2.
   a. Brachial artery (1)
   b. Following a fracture, blood vessels in the broken bone tear and haemorrhage. This results in the formation of a haematoma, at the site of the break (1)
   c. Increasing pain (½)
      Muscle tenderness and swelling (½)
      Sensory deficit of nerves passing through forearm (½)
      Prolonged capillary refill time (½)
   d. Mesenchymal stem cells (1)
   e. Correct shading of area (1)
      Anterior interosseous branch of median nerve (1)

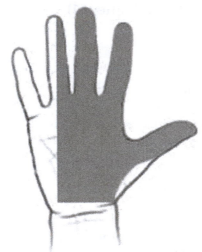

   f. Test for grip and pinch, specifically thumb, index and middle finger flexion (1)
      Test for OK sign (tests FDP and FPL) – patient will be unable to make this sign (1)
   g. This is non-union as a consequence of lacking adequate bone stability, blood flow or both. There may have been some displacement in the original fracture (or while in the cast) which prevented healing (1)

This questions focuses on supracondylar fractures, which is the most common fracture of childhood. It usually occurs as a result of a fall on a hyperextended elbow. The worrying feature of this fracture is the neuro-vascular compromise to the brachial artery, median (anterior interosseous branch), radial or ulnar nerves. In addition to neurovascular compromise, other key complications include malunion resulting in cubitus varus and ischaemic contracture (Volkmann contracture) due to brachial artery injury that results in impaired circulation leading to forearm compartment syndrome.

3.
    a. Erb-Duchenne palsy is an upper brachial plexus palsy. (1) It affects C5 and C6 roots (superior trunk) (1)
    b. Any one of the following scores one mark: total of two marks.
       Subclavian artery
       Subclavian vein
       Internal jugular vein
       Axillary artery
       Supraclavicular nerves
    c. The lateral fragment is usually pulled inferiorly by the weight of the arm (1) and medially by the pectoralis major. (1) The medial fragment tends to be displaced superiorly by the action of the sternocleidomastoid muscle (1)
    d. Any one of the following scores one mark: total of two marks.
       Protects the brachial plexus, major underlying vessels and the lung apex
       Attaches upper limb to trunk
       Transmits forces from the upper limb to the axial skeleton
    e. A pneumothorax is a potential acute complication of clavicle fractures (1)

This question focuses on clavicle fractures which usually occur secondary to a fall on to an outstretched hand or a direct blow to the shoulder. These fractures are most common in the middle third. Patients may show sagging of the shoulder downwards, and forwards an obvious deformity over the break and inability to the lift the arm. Complications included neurovascular injury especially to the brachial plexus and subclavian vessels and pneumothorax. Management is usually via a broad arm sling with follow-up X-rays at 6 weeks to ensure union.

4.
    a. Failure to abduct and place leg under torso when walking, due to obturator nerve damage causing adductor paralysis (1)
    b. Discredited condition causing enacted stigma (1)
       Social isolation, for example, due to difficulties participating in playing (1)
    c. Any one of the following scores one mark:
       Osteoarthritis due to joint instability
       Decreased mobility and instability on walking

d. Any one of the following correct answers score one mark: total of six marks.

	Major nerve	Dermatome
Hip flexion	Femoral	L2-4
Leg adduction	Obturator	L2-4
Knee flexion	Sciatic	L4-S3

This question focuses on a limping child. The most common cause is a minor injury but if there is persistent limping you must consider whether there is an underlying infection or inflammatory disease. Transient synovitis is the next most common cause of a limp after a minor injury. Other causes to consider include Perthe's disease which typically occurs between 4 and 10 years of age and slipped upper femoral epiphysis which typically affects 10 to 16-year-olds. When a child presents with a limp you must rule out septic arthritis and then consider other pathologies according to the age group, for example, tubercular arthritis typically occurring within the age group of two to five years.

5.
a. Humeral dislocation injures the axillary nerve (1) causing deltoid denervation wasting (1), revealing the contour of the underlying acromion.
b. The acromioclavicular joint (1)
c. They insert into the greater and lesser tubercle of the humerus, so they are superolateral to the glenohumeral joint (1)
d. Any one of the following scores one mark: total of two marks.
  Glenoid labrum (deepens glenoid fossa)
  Coracoacromial ligament/arch (prevents superior dislocation)
  Deltoid tone prevents inferior dislocation
  Glenohumeral ligaments
e. Supraspinatus muscle (1) up to 15–20 degrees
f. Shoulder impingement syndrome (1), also called painful arc syndrome. This occurs when the tendons of the rotator cuff muscles become irritated and inflamed as they pass under the coracoacromial arch resulting in pain, weakness and reduced range of movement at the shoulder (1)
g. Partial loss of continuity between the articular surfaces (1)

This question focuses on shoulder dislocation which is classified into anterior, posterior or inferior. Anterior dislocation is the most common and usually follows a fall on an arm or shoulder. Ensure that pulses and nerves are checked especially the axillary nerve supplying sensation over the lower deltoid area. Posterior dislocation is rare and presents with a limitation of external rotation. Inferior dislocation is rarer and usually occurs from hyperabduction. This type of dislocation has a high incidence of complications, for example, neurovascular injury, tuberosity avulsion and rotator cuff tear.

6.
  a. Anterior longitudinal ligament (1)
  b. i. Annulus fibrosus (1)
     ii. Nucleus pulposus (1)
  c. Magnetic resonance imaging (1)
  d. Lateral aspect of leg and dorsal part of foot (1)
  e. Tibialis anterior (1)
     Extensor hallucis longus (1)
  f. The spinous process does not bifurcate (1)
  g. They inhibit SNS input to bladder detrusor muscles and urethral
     sphincter (1)
     They simulate contraction of the detrusor muscles (1)

This question focuses on back pain. Local pain is deep and aching whereas
radicular pain is stabbing due to compression of dorsal nerve roots. In this
scenario, the patient presents with disc prolapse. Lumbar discs are most
likely to rupture especially L4/L5 and L5/S1. When pain radiates to the
leg this is termed sciatica. Signs are dependent on the nerve compressed,
for example, in L4/L5 prolapse the L5 root will be compressed and you
would expect weak hallux extension and decreased sensation on the
outer dorsum of the foot. One emergency that must be ruled out is cauda
equina compression which presents with decreased saddle-area sensation,
incontinence/retention of faeces or urine, poor anal tone and paralysis with
or without sensory loss.

7.
  a. Any one of the following scores one mark: total of two marks.
     Immobility
     Mental confusion
     Reduced reaction times, sensory perception, proprioception
     Impaired compensatory blood pressure mechanisms
     Polypharmacy
  b. The affected leg may be externally rotated, adducted and shortened (1)
  c. Any one of the following scores one mark: all three correct for two
     marks.
     Medial circumflex femoral artery
     Lateral circumflex femoral artery
     Artery of ligamentum teres
  d. i. An intracapsular fracture is within the fibrous articular capsule of the
        hip joint, commonly a femoral neck fracture. An extracapsular fracture
        is outside the fibrous articular capsule of the hip joint, commonly an
        intertrochanteric or subtrochanteric fracture (1)
     ii. Prognostic value and management is different. Disruption of the
        blood supply to the femoral head frequently occurs and can lead to
        avascular necrosis. Intracapsular fractures need internal fixation
        with screws or arthroplasty. Extracapsular fractures may require
        extramedullary hip screws or intramedullary nails (1)

    e. Osteoporosis is a condition that is characterised by a decrease in bone mass and density, causing bones to become fragile. (1) It is more common in elderly women due to the reduction in oestrogen after menopause. Oestrogen is protective as it stimulates osteoblast activity and inhibits osteoclast activity (1)

    f. Any one of the following scores half a mark: total of one mark

    Rapid functional decline

    Increased risk of infection (e.g. MRSA)

    Mental confusion

    Other complications related to immobility (DVT, pressure sores)

    Financial/employment issues

This question focuses on hip fractures. These can be classified into intracapsular or extracapsular fractures. Intracapsular fractures occur just below the femoral head and patients usually present with an externally rotated, adducted and shortened hip. Avascular necrosis of the head can occur as the medial femoral circumflex artery supplies the head via the neck. Extracapsular fractures occur between the greater and lesser trochanters. With these fractures there is adequate blood supply so malunion is rarer.

8.

    a. The most common mechanism of injury for all types of wrist fractures is a fall on an outstretched hand (FOOSH). (1) The wrist is hyperextended and the point of impact causes energy forces through the distal radius that result in various fractures (1)

    b. Any one of the following scores half a mark: total of one mark.

    Poor blood supply

    Patient age

    Excessive mobility

    Infection

    Smoking

    Malnutrition

    c. Any one of the following scores one mark: total of two marks.

    Deformity

    Arthritis

    Chronic pain

    Malunion/non-union

    Nerve damage

    d. A fracture arising within weakened/abnormal bone due to another disease process (1)

    e. Most commonly, the scaphoid breaks in its mid-portion, known as the 'waist' (1)

    f. An X-ray (1)

    g. Avascular necrosis of proximal segment. (1) This is because of the blood supply to the scaphoid which is distal to proximal (1)

This question focuses on distal radial fractures, for example, Colles' fracture. This type of fracture is common in osteoporotic postmenopausal women who fall on an outstretched hand. Patients usually present with a 'dinner-fork' deformity of the wrist as a result of dorsal angulation and displacement. On X-ray the injury comprises a transverse fracture of the distal radius with dorsal displacement and shortening of the wrist. A ulnar styloid fracture usually occurs with a Colles' fracture. Other types of distal radial fractures include Smith's fracture, Barton's fracture and scaphoid fractures.

9.

    a. Femoral vein (1)

    b. Anteromedial thigh (1)

       Medial side of leg and foot (1)

    c. Tibial nerve (1) L4–S3 (1)

    d. Any correct answer scores half a mark: total of two marks.

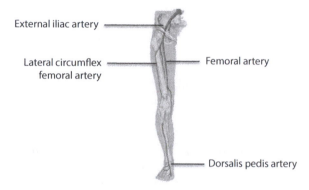

    e. Superior – inguinal ligament (1)

       Medial – medial border of adductor longus muscle (1)

       Lateral – medial border of sartorius muscle (1)

This question focuses on the anatomy of the femoral triangle, an area within the anterior thigh. The femoral triangle has three borders: the superior, lateral and medial. In addition, the anterior (roof) border of the triangle is formed by the fascia lata and the posterior (base) is formed by the pectineus, iliopsoas and adductor longus muscle. Many neurovascular structures lie within the triangle which include, from lateral to medial, the femoral nerve, femoral artery, femoral vein and femoral canal, of which the artery, vein and canal are contained within the femoral sheath.

MCQ

1. C

This scenario describes a psoas abscess. The psoas muscle is covered by the psoas fascia, a sheath that is open superiorly therefore allowing infection around the soft tissues of the spine to enter and spread to the groin. The sartorius, rectus femoris and vastus lateralis are muscles of the anterior thigh compartment therefore not in relation to the lumbar spine. The gluteus minimus is one of the muscles that makes up the buttocks and therefore not related to the groin.

2. E

This scenario describes carpal tunnel syndrome, a condition due to compression of the median nerve as it travels through the carpal tunnel at the wrist. Hence, patients will present with signs and symptoms associated with median nerve functions. This would result in reduced sensation to the lateral part of the palm and lateral three and a half fingers on the palmar surface of the hand. In addition, the thenar muscles and lateral two lumbricals would be affected resulting in loss of co-ordination and strength of the thumb and flexion, and extension of index and middle fingers at the metacarpophalangeal and interphalangeal joints, respectively. Option (a) describes damage to the radial nerve, option (b) is damage to the ulnar nerve, option (c) is damage to the adductor pollicis and option (d) is damage to the extensor pollicis brevis.

3. B

Most commonly in a shoulder dislocation the humerus exits the joint inferiorly where the joint capsule is the weakest. The axillary nerve is formed within the axilla region and travels through the quadrangular space with the posterior circumflex humeral artery. The axillary nerve is most commonly damaged by trauma to the shoulder or proximal humerus.

4. A

The gluteus medius and minimus are the two muscles that abduct and medially rotate the lower limb. These muscles secure the pelvis preventing the drop of the pelvis of the opposite limb. The superior gluteal nerve innervates both muscles and damage to this nerve classically presents with trendelenburg gait.

5. C

All compounds listed can produce crystals. Monosodium urate crystals that are negatively birefringent under polarised light microscopy confirms diagnosis of gout. Pseudogout reveals positive birefringent calcium pyrophosphate under polarised light microscopy. Calcium phosphate crystals are associated with osteoarthritis and cholesterol crystals are seen in inflammatory and degenerative arthritis.

6. B

Erb's palsy is due to the damage of the brachial plexus usually to the fifth and sixth cervical nerve. The brachial plexus is a network of nerves consisting of C5-T1 that supplies the skin and musculature of the upper limb. This plexus is divided into roots, trunks, divisions, cords and branches. The roots are formed by the nerves C5-T1. The superior trunk is a combination of C5 and C6, the middle trunk is a continuation of C7 and the inferior trunk is a combination of C8 and T1. Each trunk is divided into anterior or posterior and the cords consist of lateral, posterior or medial. Finally there are five major branches consisting of musculocutaneous, axillary, median, radial and ulnar nerves.

7. D

The anatomical snuffbox is a triangular deepening found on the lateral aspect of the dorsum of the hand. The borders include the ulnar (medial) formed by tendon of extensor pollicis longus, radial (lateral) formed by the tendons of abductor pollicis longus and extensor pollicis brevis and proximal border formed by the styloid process of the radius.

EMQ

This question is based on the various nerves of the upper limb

8. F

This is a classic presentation of posterior interosseous nerve compression. Patients typically complain of proximal forearm pain with partial to complete motor paralysis of wrist extension. Patients will be unable to extend a thumb or other digits at the metacarpophalangeal joints as the majority of extensor muscles and abductor pollicis longus muscle are affected.

9. D

A positive Froment's sign indicates ulnar nerve palsy. The small muscles of the hand will be paralysed except for muscles of thenar eminence and the first two lumbricals. Consequently, the patient is unable to adduct and abduct fingers and unable to grip a piece of paper between the fingers.

10. C

The suprascapular nerve innervates both the supraspinatus and infraspinatus muscles. Therefore, paralysis of this nerve will cause problems with abduction and external rotation of the humerus and wasting of both muscles.

Reproductive System (Chapter 12)

1.

    a. Labelling of each correct element scores one mark: total of two marks.
       (Seminiferous tubules are circles, and Leydig cells surround them)

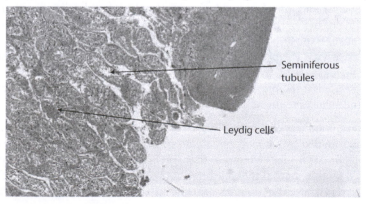

   b. The luteinising hormone binds to Leydig cells (1)
      The follicle-stimulating hormone binds to Sertoli cells (1)
   c. Leydig cell and lutenising hormone binding leads to increased testosterone synthesis (1)
      Sertoli cell and follicle-stimulating hormone binding leads to spermatogenesis (1)
   d. This is a continuation of the tail of epididymis and runs in the spermatic cord through the inguinal canal. (1) It travels through the sidewall of the pelvis close to the ischial tuberosity, travels medially and joints with ducts from the seminal vesicle to form the ejaculatory duct which joins the prostatic urethra inferiorly to the bladder (1)
   e. Pigmented skin, dartos fascia, external spermatic fascia, cremaster fascia, internal spermatic fascia, tunica vaginalis, testes (2)

This question focuses on the histology of the male reproductive tract. This consists of the testis, duct system (efferent ducts, epididymis, vas deferens) and glands (seminal vesicle, prostate). The seminiferous epithelium consists of two cell types, the Sertoli cells and cells of the germ cell lineage. The Sertoli cells are responsive to follicle-stimulating hormone and secrete inhibin. The Leydig cells are responsible for testosterone secretion. Tumours of the testis are very important with a high proportion seen in early life. Between 90% and 95% of testicular neoplasms are germ cell tumours.

2.
   a. i. Fibroadenoma (½)
         Cyst (½)
      ii. Fibrocystic disease (½)
          Adenocarcinoma (½)
   b. Medial aspect drains into parasternal and opposite breast (1)
      Lateral aspect drains into the axillary lymph nodes (1)
   c. Oestrogen is responsible for the proliferation of the duct system (1)
      Progesterone leads to development of secretory tissue (1)
   d. The lack of placenta after delivery leads to an abrupt decrease in oestrogen and progesterone levels (1)
   e. The production of steroid hormones by the ovary begins at around the time of menarche and decreases rapidly at around the time of menopause. Exposure to these is a risk factor for breast cancer (1)
   f. Sensitivity: the proportion of people who have the disease and test positive for it (1)
      Specificity: the proportion of people who test positive for the disease and who have the actual disease (1)

This question focuses on breast disease. The breast is composed of mammary glands surrounded by a connective tissue stroma. Arterial supply to the medial part of the breast is via the internal thoracic artery. The lateral part of the breast is supplied by the internal thoracic and thoracoacromial branches (from the axillary artery), lateral mammary branches (from posterior intercostal arteries) and the mammary branch (from the anterior intercostal artery). Lymphatic drainage of the lateral quadrants of the breast drains to axillary lymph nodes whereas the medial quadrants of the breast drain to the parasternal nodes or to the opposite breast. Fibrocystic changes, such as cysts, apocrine metaplasia and fibrosis, are related to the imbalance between oestrogen and progesterone due to anovulation and therefore more common towards the age of menopause. Benign tumours include fibroadenoma (commonest benign tumour, mainly occurring in young women), ductal papilloma, adenoma, connective tissue tumours and benign phyllodes tumours. Breast cancer is the commonest tumour in women and can be classified into in situ carcinoma (ductal, lobular) and invasive carcinoma.

3.
   a. Any one of the following scores one mark: total of four marks.
      Ultrasound scan (20 weeks): amniotic fluid volume, size, date of pregnancy, gross deformities, placenta praevia
      Bloods: alpha-foetoprotein, iron, folate
      Symphysis-fundal height
      Maternal urine: protein, leucocytes/nitrites, glucose
      Amniocentesis (may need specialist clinic)
   b. Foetal alcohol syndrome causes mental retardation, head and neck deformities. (1) This occurs because ethanol is lipid soluble and diffuses freely across the placenta (1)
   c. Pregnancy-induced hypertension in association with proteinuria with or without oedema (1)
   d. Any one of the following scores half a mark: total of one mark.
      Headache
      Chest or epigastric pain
      Vomiting
      Visual disturbance
      Hyperreflexia
      Irritability
   e. Any one of the following scores one mark: total of two marks.
      Knowledge does not necessarily empower people (fallacy of empowerment)
      Can promote victim blaming
      Cultural issues

This question focuses on the various medical conditions related to pregnancy. Antenatal care aims to detect any disease in the mother, prepare mothers for birth, monitor trends to prevent or detect any early complications of pregnancy and ameliorate discomforts of pregnancy. At the booking appointment (by 10 weeks) a variety of checks are undertaken, for example, general (height, weight, BMI, blood pressure), urinalysis and booking bloods. Other tests such as screening for Down's syndrome occur at specific weeks of gestation. Subsequent checks occur at various stages throughout pregnancy. High levels of alcohol consumption are known to cause foetal alcohol syndrome and features include microcephaly, short palpebral fissure, hypoplastic upper lip, absent philtrum, small eyes and cardiac malformations. Pre-eclampsia is essentially pregnancy-induced hypertension with proteinuria with or without oedema. The main defect is the failure of trophoblast invasion of spiral arteries therefore leaving them vasoactive.

4.
  a. Any one of the following scores one mark: total of two marks.
    Stress
    Weight loss
    Increase exercise
    Polycystic ovarian syndrome
    Thyroid disease
    Pregnancy
  b. Any one of the following score half a mark: total of three marks.

Day	Oestrogen	Progesterone
7	Rising	Low
14	High	Rising
21	Low	High

  c. Progesterone stimulates appetite and diverts glucose into fat synthesis. (1)
  d. Human placental lactogen generates a maternal resistance to insulin therefore decreases maternal glucose usage (1) and increases lipolysis. (1)
  e. Any one of the following scores one mark: total of two marks.
    Alpha-fetoprotein
    Beta HCG
    Inhibin A
    Oestriol

This question focuses on amenorrhoea and the menstrual cycle. Primary amenorrhoea is defined as the failure to establish menstruation by the age of 16 years or by 14 years of age if no secondary sexual characteristics. Secondary amenorrhoea is defined as the absence of menstruation for six or more consecutive months in a woman who has previously established regular menses. Causes of primary amenorrhoea include constitutional delay, androgen insensitivity syndrome, anatomical defects, Kallmann syndrome, anorexia nervosa and excessive exercise. Secondary amenorrhoea causes include pregnancy, polycystic ovarian syndrome, premature ovarian failure and hypopituitarism. The menstrual cycle is co-ordinated by gonadotropins and gonadal steroids (oestrogen, progesterone). The gonadotropins act on the follicular phase where follicle-stimulating hormone (FSH) binds to the granulosa cells and the lutenising hormone (LH) binds to theca cells. This phase is to stimulate the development of the follicle. During pre-ovulation LH surge occurs to stimulate ovulation. During the luteal phase LH maintains the corpus luteum. Oestrogen during the follicular phase has many actions, for example, stimulating fallopian tube function, thickening of endometrium and thin alkaline cervical mucus. Also during the luteal phase, progesterone acts on the oestrogen-primed cells to cause further thickening of endometrium into a secretory form, thickening of myometrium and a thick, acid cervical mucus. At the beginning of the cycle, oestrogen and progesterone levels are low and FSH levels rise. During mid-follicular phase oestrogen levels are rising, inhibin levels are rising and LH levels rise. After ovulation the corpus luteum forms spontaneously and beings to secrete progesterone and oestrogen thereby maintaining suppression of FSH and LH. During the luteal phase the corpus luteum grows and secretes more steroids but after 14 days precisely it dies causing a rapid fall in steroid levels and stimulates menses (start of new cycle).

5.
   a. i. Foetal crown-rump length (1)
       ii. Foetal biometry (biparietal diameter and head circumference) (1)
   b. The top of the uterus to the top of the pubic symphysis (1)
   c. Amniotic fluid is formed from maternal plasma, and passes through the foetal membranes by osmotic and hydrostatic forces. When foetal kidneys begin to function at around 16 weeks, foetal urine also contributes to the fluid. (1) Amniotic fluid is swallowed and absorbed through the skin of the foetus (1)
   d. Polyhydramnios (1)
   e. Any one of the following scores one mark:
      Jejunum
      Ileum
      Colon
      Oesophageal
      Biliary
      Atresia occurs if recanalisation is wholly or partially unsuccessful (1)
   f. Any one of the following scores one mark: total of two marks.
      Idiopathic
      Failure of foetal swallowing (neurological, chromosomal anomalies)
      Foetal gastrointestinal tract abnormality (oesophageal atresia)
      Congenital infections
      Foetal polyuria (diabetes)

This question focuses on foetal physiology. The foetus makes breathing movements 1–4 hours each day. It also flushes the lungs with amniotic fluid. Amniotic fluid surrounds the foetus and acts as a mechanical protection, and provides a moist environment. There is about 10 ml produced at 8 weeks rising to one litre at 38 weeks then it falls to 300 ml at 42 weeks. During early pregnancy the fluid is formed from maternal fluids and from foetal extracellular fluid by diffusion across non-keratinised skin. Later in pregnancy the turnover of amniotic fluid is via the foetus. Amniotic fluid contains cells from both foetus and amnion, in addition to a variety of proteins, therefore it is very useful as a diagnostic tool (amniocentesis). Amniotic fluid abnormalities include polyhydramnios which is associated with oesophageal/duodenal atresia causing an inability to swallow amniotic fluid and with anencephaly. Oligohydramnios is associated with bilateral renal agenesis or posterior urethral valves (males) and resulting in an inability to excrete urine.

6.

    a. Menopause occurs due to ovarian failure associated with a dramatic decline in oocytes (1) and a reduction in ovarian sensitivity to gonadotropins (1)

    b. Stratum functionalis of the endometrium layer of the uterine lining (1)
       Correct labelling of stratum functionalis layer (1)
       Other labels are for reference only.

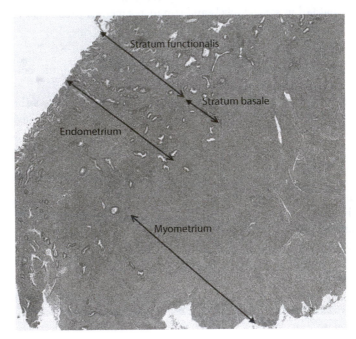

    c. Oestrogen stimulates regeneration of the stratum functionalis of the endometrium during the proliferative phase. It causes marked proliferation of endometrial stroma (1) and endometrial glands (1)

    d. Excess adipose tissue contains high levels of aromatase, an enzyme involved in the biosynthesis of oestrogen from androgens. (1) Therefore, a higher BMI results in a greater amount of oestrogen thereby inducing endometrial proliferation (1)

    e. Hysterectomy performed to remove and stage the tumour. (1) A bilateral salpingo-oophrectomy is performed to exclude the possibility of hormone producing a tumour in the ovaries (1)

This question focuses on menopause and gynaecological tumours. The menopause is the cessation of menstrual cycles, which occurs at an average of between 49 and 50 years of age. At this stage no follicles develop and oestrogen levels fall dramatically. FSH and LH levels rise with a dramatic rise in FSH due to no inhibin production. Endometrial carcinoma is a cancer of the uterine body that usually presents as postmenopausal bleeding. The majority are adenocarcinomas and are related to excessive exposure to oestrogen unopposed by progesterone. Risk factors include obesity, nullipara, early menarche and late menopause.

7.
    a. Fitz-Hugh–Curtis syndrome. (1) It is a type of perihepatitis that causes liver capsular infection and inflammation with adhesions, producing right upper quadrant pain due to the transabdominal spread of infection (1)

    b. Right and left paracolic gutters and right and left paramesenteric gutters. (1) These recesses allow a passage for infectious fluids from different compartments of the abdomen (1)

    c. Any one of the following scores half a mark: total of one mark.
       Purulent vaginal discharge
       Abnormal vaginal bleeding (postcoital, intermenstrual or menorrhagia)
       Deep dyspareunia

    d. Neisseria gonorrhoeae and Chlamydia trachomatis (1)

    e. Endocervical swabs for C. trachomatis and N. gonorrhoeae (1)

    f. Urinalysis (1)

    g. Any one of the following scores one mark: total of two marks.
       Increased risk of future ectopic pregnancy
       Tubal infertility
       Chronic pelvic pain

This question focuses on genital tract infections. Genital skin and mucous membrane lesions can present as genital ulcers, vesicles or bullae, genital papules or anogenital warts. Patients who present with urethritis (discharge, dysuria, frequency) could be as a result of gonococcal urethritis, chlamydial urethritis, post-gonococcal urethritis or non-infectious urethritis. Common pathogens of sexually transmitted infections (STIs) include human papillomaviruses, herpes simplex virus types one and two, C. trachomatis, N. gonorrhoeae, T. vaginalis and T. pallidum. Pelvic inflammatory disease is a result of ascending infections of the genital tract (endometritis, salpingitis, tubo-ovarian abscess). It is commonly caused by STIs (often chlamydia and gonorrhoeae). In acute cases patients present with bilateral lower abdominal pain, vaginal discharge, fever, irregular vaginal bleed and dyspareunia.

8.
    a. Any one of the following scores one mark: total of three marks.
       Foetal heart rate
       Foetal breathing
       Foetal movement

Foetal tone
Amniotic fluid volume
b. At 18 weeks the lung is in the canalicular phase of development. Gas exchange surfaces are not yet developed, therefore a foetus would not be viable. (1) Surfactant is a phospholipid that causes a reduction in the surface tension of the alveolus. (1) It is produced by type II alveolar cells, which, although they are present from an early stage in foetal development, do not start to produce surfactant until closer to term in the saccular phase of development. This begins from about 24 weeks (1)
c. Asymmetrical intrauterine growth restriction is a type of growth restriction (IUGR) where the abdominal circumference is disproportion-ately smaller than the head (1)
Placental insufficiency is a common cause (1)
d. Oxytocin activates phospholipase C to produce inositol 1,4,5-trisphos-phate, which releases calcium from intracellular stores. This stimulates myometrial contractions in labour (1)
e. Sacrovertebral angle to pubis symphysis (1)

This question focuses on foetal growth and development. Antenatal assessment of foetal well-being includes foetal movements, measurements of uterine expansion (symphysis-fundal height) and an ultrasound scan. An ultrasound scan is routinely carried out at approximately 20 weeks to assess foetal growth and foetal anomalies. The crown-rump length is measured between 7 and 13 weeks to date the pregnancy and estimate the delivery date. Biparietal diameter (BPD) is the distance between the parietal bones of the foetal skull and is used in combination with other measurements to date pregnancies in trimesters two and three. Abdominal circumference and femur length in combination with BPD is used for dating and growth monitoring, and can be used to detect any anomalies.

9.
a. This is 84% or approximately 8 in 10 (1)
b. Any one of the following scores half a mark: total of one mark.
Polycystic ovarian syndrome
Hypogonadotropic hypogonadism
Premature ovarian failure
Pituitary tumours
Hyperprolactinaemia
c. Sperm count of <15 million/ml is regarded too low for reliable fertility. (1)
Normal volume of ejaculate is >1.5ml (1)
d. Progressive motility (1) and sperm morphology (1)
e. Human chorionic gonadotropin (1)
f. Human chorionic gonadotropin (hCG) is synthesised primarily by the villous syncytiotrophoblast. (1) Peak levels are reached at 8–10 weeks. (1) hCG maintains maternal corpus luteum that secretes progesterone

and oestrogens before placental production replaces this by the end of the first trimester (1)

This question focuses on infertility. This is defined as failure to conceive following at least 1 year of regular unprotected sexual intercourse. This can be either primary (no previous pregnancy) or secondary (previous pregnancy). Causes can be due to coital problems, anovulation (15%–20%), tubal occlusion (15%–40%) and abnormal/absent sperm production (20%–25%). Causes of anovulation can be due to hyperprolactinaemia, weight loss, exercise, stress, pituitary tumours, ovarian failure and polycystic ovarian syndrome. Tubal occlusion can be caused by sterilisation and scarring from infection and endometriosis. Absent sperm production can be due to abnormal production (e.g. testicular disease), obstruction of ducts (e.g. infection, vasectomy) and hypothalamic/pituitary dysfunction.

10.

    a. Adplantation of blastocyst on to endometrium – following hatching from the zona pellucida on Day 5. This first phase requires the newly hatched blastocyst to loosely adhere to the endometrial epithelium, often 'rolling' to the eventual site of implantation (1)
Adhesion of blastocyst on to endometrium – the microvilli on the surface of the outermost trophoblast cells interact with the epithelial cells of the uterus through cell surface glycoproteins (1)
Invasion of trophoblast and embedding – the trophoblast differentiates into the outer syncytiotrophoblast and the inner cytotrophoblast. The syncytiotrophoblast produces lytic enzymes and penetrates into the stroma that lie below (1)

    b. The ampulla of the fallopian tube (1)

    c. Any one of the following scores half a mark: total of one mark.
Pelvic inflammatory disease
Sexually transmitted infection
Previous tubal surgery
Previous ectopic pregnancy

    d. Ruptured ectopic pregnancy leading to hypovolaemic shock (1)

    e. In response to the blood loss there is inadequate circulating volume. There is subsequent inadequate organ perfusion and failure, and blood pressure falls. Compensatory mechanisms are activated when baroreceptors sense the fall in blood pressure and cause the release of nor-adrenaline and adrenaline. (1) Noradrenaline causes predominantly vasoconstriction and a slight increase in heart rate. (1) Adrenaline predominantly causes an increase in heart rate with a slight increase in vascular tone. (1) The overall effect is an increase in blood pressure. Sweat and cold hands are due to activation of this sympathetic nervous system resulting in vasoconstriction (1)

This question focuses on ectopic pregnancy. This is when pregnancy occurs outside the uterus, usually in the fallopian tubes mainly within the ampullary region.

However, it can also occur in the ovary, uterus, broad ligament and abdomen. Associated risks include sexually transmitted infection/pelvic inflammatory disease, previous tubal surgery, previous ectopic pregnancy and assisted conception. Patients typically present with abdominal pain, amenorrhoea with or without vaginal bleeding, shoulder tip pain and dizziness. It is important to note that a ruptured ectopic pregnancy may present with circulatory collapse. Complications include rupture, haemorrhage, tubal infertility and death.

MCQ

1. A

The foetus has two duct systems, the Müllerian (paramesonephric) duct and the Wolffian (mesonephric) duct. The Müllerian duct forms the female internal genitalia (ovaries, fallopian tube, uterus, cervix, vagina) whereas the Wolffian duct forms the male internal genitalia (epididymis, vas deferens, seminal vesicles, prostate gland, bulbourethral glands).

2. D

Chlamydia trachomatis can be isolated in up to 50% of women with gonorrhoea. Patients treated for gonorrhoea may go on to develop chlamydia or pelvic inflammatory disease. Therefore any patients treated for gonorrhoea should also be treated for chlamydia either with azithromycin or doxycycline.

3. D

The contents of the greater sciatic foramen include seven nerves (sciatic, superior gluteal, inferior gluteal, posterior femoral cutaneous, pudendal nerve, nerve to quadratus femoris, nerve to obturator internus), three vessels (superior gluteal artery and vein, inferior gluteal and vein, internal pudendal artery and vein) and one muscle (piriformis). The lesser sciatic foramen contents include the tendon of the obturator internus, pudendal nerve, internal pudendal vessels and nerve to the obturator internus.

4. E

This scenario describes endometrial cancer. Most are adenocarcinomas and related to excessive exposure to oestrogen unopposed by progesterone. It usually presents as postmenopausal bleeding. Risk factors include obesity, unopposed oestrogen, nulliparity and late menopause.

5. B

Sperm is produced in the testes and when ejaculation occurs it is expelled from the tail of epididymis into the vas deferens. Sperm then travels through the vas deferens through up the spermatic cord into the pelvic cavity over the ureter to the prostate behind the bladder. Vas deferens then joins the seminal vesicle to form an ejaculatory duct which passes through the prostate and empties into the urethra.

6. E

Lymphatic drainage of the vulva is to the superficial inguinal lymph nodes. Structures of the vulva include the mon pubis, labia majora, labia minora, vestibule, Bartholin's glands and clitoris.

7. C

According to the WHO classification, below are the parameters for semen analysis:

Volume	1.5 ml
Sperm concentration	15×10^6 spermatozoa/ml
Motility	32%
Morphology	4% normally formed

EMQ

This question is based on the menstrual cycle

8. H

The spiral arteries of the functional layer are hormone sensitive and constrict when the progesterone concentration decreases. These contractions of the spiral arteries are responsible for an interruption of blood supply therefore cells die leading to menstruation.

9. B

Lutenising hormone surge occurs on Day 13 and lasts for 24–48 hours. This surge triggers ovulation by releasing the egg from the follicle and converts residual follicle into corpus luteum which produces progesterone ready for implantation.

10. E

Theca interna cells express receptors for lutenising hormone to produce androgen. Granulosa cells convert these androgens to oestrogen.

Neurology (Chapter 13)

1.
   a. Left. (1) The contralateral hemisphere supplies motor and sensation, due to decussation (1)
   b. Thromboembolic stroke (1)
      Haemorrhagic stroke (1)
   c. It is produced in the choroid plexus via ultrafiltration in the ventricles, travels via interventricular foramen (Monro) from lateral to third ventricle, through the cerebral aqueduct into the fourth ventricle, via the foramina of Magendie and Luschka into subarachnoid space (1) and reabsorbed via the arachnoid granulations in the superior Saggital sinus (1)

    d. i. C5–C6 (1)
        ii. S1 (1)
        iii. L3–L4 (1)
    e. Hypertonia (spasticity) in right arm whereas left arm will be normal (1)

2.

    a. Long-term alcohol abuse results in degeneration of neurones in the cerebellar cortex via nutritional deficiency which are important for nervous system function (1)
    b. Alcohol is oxidised to acetaldehyde via alcohol dehydrogenase (1) Acetaldehyde is then oxidised to acetate via aldehyde dehydrogenase (1)
    c. Any one of the following scores half a mark: total of three marks.
        A – Thalamus
        B – Hypothalamus
        C – Midbrain
        D – Pons
        E – Corpus callosum
        F – Cerebellum
    d. Dysmetria, dysdiadochokinesia and ataxia (1)
    e. When a peripheral nerve is transected, Wallerian degeneration of distal axons begins. (1) Macrophages, phagocytes and Schwann cells then migrate to area of injury to clear necrotic debris. (1) Axonal sprouting then occurs at the proximal stump and grows until they enter the distal stump (1)

The first two questions focus on some general neurology knowledge. Note the nerve roots for the reflex arcs which are commonly tested during a neurological examination. Knowledge of the anatomy of the brain and what different areas of the brain may be involved with in terms of functions is important when thinking about different neurological diseases.

3.

    a. Any one of the following scores one mark: all three for two marks.
        Problems initiating movement
        Festinating gait (stooped, short steps, decreased arm movement)
        Problems altering movement (turning and stopping)
    b. Any one of the following scores one mark: total of two marks.
        Pill-rolling tremor (resting)
        Masked facies
        Micrographia
        Postural instability
        Cog-wheel or lead pipe rigidity
    c. Basal ganglia (1) are composed of the striatum (caudate and putamen) and globus pallidus (called lentiform nucleus along with putamen). They are sub-cortical nuclei that are separated from the thalamus by the internal capsule, and they lie under the insular lobe (1)

Any one of the following scores one mark: total of two marks.
Functions include:
Control of voluntary motor activity
Control of reflex muscular activity
Control of muscle tone

d. Any one of the following scores one mark: total of two marks.
Levodopa – crosses blood brain barrier and taken up dopaminergic cells in substantia nigra where it is converted to dopamine by dopa-decarboxylase
Dopamine agonists – bind to dopaminergic post-synaptic receptors in brain
Monoamine B inhibitors – increase level of dopamine in basal ganglia by blocking its metabolism
Apomorphine – a potent dopamine agonist
COMT inhibitors – reversibly inhibit the peripheral breakdown of levodopa by the COMT enzyme therefore increasing the amount for conversion to dopamine

This question focuses on Parkinson's disease (PD), which is caused by degeneration of the dopaminergic pathways in the substantia nigra. Onset is gradual and insidious with a peak age of 55–65. It is characterised by tremor at rest, rigidity and bradykinesia. Other types of Parkinsonism to be aware of are the 'atypical' or 'parkinson plus' syndromes. They are similar to PD but more severe with a median survival of around 7 years. They include:

- Multiple system atrophy – characterised by early autonomic features, often with a poor or temporary response to levodopa therapy.
- Progressive supranuclear palsy – characterised by paresis of conjugate gaze, initially with problems with vertical gaze.

4.

a. Any one of the following scores one mark: total of two marks.
Papilloedema
Esotropia
Mydriasis
Ptosis

b. Any one of the following haemorrhages with description scores two marks: total of four marks.
Extradural – potential space between skull and periosteal dura, due to meningeal artery rupture
Subarachnoid – actual space between arachnoid and pia mater containing cerebrospinal fluid Spontaneous bleeding into subarachnoid space commonly due to rupture of saccular aneurysms
Subdural – potential space between dura and arachnoid, due to rupture of the bridging veins

c. Cerebrospinal fluid otorrhoea (1)

d. Temporal bone (petrous part containing inner ear) (1)

e. Facial (1) and vestibulocochlear (1)

This question is looking at potential intercranial injuries. It is important to be aware of the intercranial haemorrhages listed above and how they may appear on CT scans. CT is very sensitive in diagnosing haemorrhage in patients in the acute stage of a cerebrovascular event. Anticoagulants should not be started until brain imaging has excluded haemorrhage.

5.
    a. Anterior spinothalamic – crude touch (1)
       Lateral spinothalamic – pain and temperature (1)

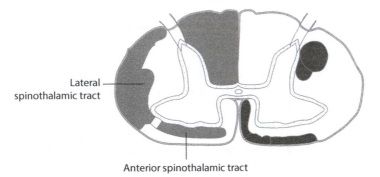

Lateral spinothalamic tract

Anterior spinothalamic tract

    b. These pathways decussate at the spinal cord and therefore correspond to the contralateral (opposite) side of the body (1)
    c. The lateral corticospinal tract decussates at the medulla and would therefore correspond to the ipsilateral side (1)
       Correct labelling as below (1)

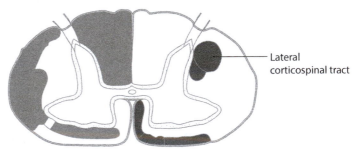

Lateral corticospinal tract

    d. This describes Brown-Sequard syndrome therefore the lesion is on the right side (1)
    e. There is no left sided plantar reflex due to loss of pain sensation on this side (1)
    f. Upper motor neurone lesion (1)
    g. Lower motor neurone (½)
       Any one of the following scores half a mark:
       Flaccid paralysis
       Hyporeflexia
       Atrophy of muscles

    h. An MRI is better suited for examining soft tissue injury and cord compromise (1)

The focus of this question is around sensory and motor tracts of the nervous system. Ascending tracts are sensory while descending tracts are motor. The three main sensory tracts are the dorsal/posterior column tract, the spinothalamic tract and the spinocerebellar tract. The dorsal column delivers fine touch, proprioception and vibration information. The spinothalamic tract delivers pain and temperature sensations. The spinocerebellar tract transmits proprioception to the cerebellum. The major descending tract to be aware of is the corticospinal tract which delivers conscious control of skeletal muscle.

6.

    a. Atherothromboembolism from carotid (1)
    b. To prevent a stroke or recurrent transient ischaemic attack (1)
    c. Antiplatelet (1)
    d. CT scan (1)
    e. Broca's aphasia (1)
    f. Inferior frontal gyrus (1)
    g. Middle cerebral artery (1)
    h. The embolism passed (1)
    i. Must not drive for 1 month (1)
       There is no need to notify DVLA after a single TIA. Multiple TIAs over a short period require 3 months free from further attacks before resuming driving and DVLA should be notified (1)

A **transient ischaemic attack** is a transient and reversible inadequacy of the circulation in part of the brain (a cerebral or retinal deficit) that gives a clinical picture similar to a stroke. The duration is no more than 24 hours. Longer than this is defined as a stroke.

7.

    a. Any one of the following scores half a mark: total of two marks.
       Loss of attention
       Loss of abstract thought
       Perseveration
       Change of affect, for example, inappropriate sexual behaviour
       Decreased lack of spontaneous activity
       Executive impairment
    b. Damage to basal ganglia (1)
    c. Atherosclerosis (1)
    d. Abnormal accumulation of cerebrospinal fluid in the ventricular system (1) of the brain with an increase in the size of ventricle, (1) hence there is no increase in the pressure within the ventricles.
    e. Gait disturbance (1)
       Sphincter disturbance (urinary and sometimes bowel incontinence) (1)
       Dementia (1)
    f. Insertion of cerebrospinal fluid shunt (1)

Normal pressure hydrocephalus (NPH) describes the ventricular dilatation in the absence of raised CSF pressure on lumbar puncture. It is characterised by a triad of gait abnormality, urinary (usually) incontinence and dementia. This dementia may be potentially reversible. **Neuroimaging** may show ventricular enlargement out of proportion to sulcal atrophy and periventricular lucency.

8.

a. Crescent-shaped haematoma suggestive of subdural haemorrhage (1)
b. Between the dura mater and arachnoid mater meningeal layers (1)
c. Bridging veins between dura and arachnoid mater. (1) These veins drain into dural venous sinus which empty into the internal jugular vein (1)
d. Lucid interval (1)
e. Any one of the following scores one mark: total of two marks.
Elderly people are more prone to falls.
The brain atrophies with age therefore making bridging veins more vulnerable.
Anticoagulant medication is more common in the elderly population.
f. Any one of the following scores one mark:
Irrigation/evacuation, for example, via burr twist drill and burr hole craniostomy
Craniotomy
g. Cerebellar tonsils are forced through the foramen magnum due to increased intercranial pressure. (1) There may be eventual compression of the brainstem therefore causing dysfunction of the centres in the brain responsible for controlling cardiac and respiratory function (1)

This question again focuses on intercranial bleeds, potential management and complications. Please see question above.

Two paired arteries are responsible for the blood supply to the brain – the **vertebral arteries,** and the **internal carotid arteries.** The terminal branches of these eventually anastomose to form a circular blood vessel called the **circle of Willis.**

A disturbance in the blood supply to the brain may lead to a stroke (or TIA). The four main causes of this are:

- Thrombus – obstruction of a blood vessel by a locally forming clot
- Emboli – obstruction due to an embolus formed elsewhere: this is the most common cause
- Haemorrhage – blood accumulates within the cranial cavity
- Hypoperfusion – lack of blood supply may be due to low blood pressure

MCQ

1. C

The length constant is the distance from the point of origin where the change in membrane potential is equal to 37% of the maximum potential change. The longer the length constant, the further the current can spread, allowing action potentials to propagate faster. Increasing membrane resistance and deceasing internal resistance of the axon can increase length constant.

2. A

Embolisation from infective endocarditis usually causes small parietal lobe abscesses. Frontal lobe is not as common as parietal lobe for septic emboli. The cerebellum is often affected in alcoholism and is not a common site for septic emboli.

3. E

This is describing déjà vu, which is a sensation that an event or experience is familiar even though it has never been previously experienced. Jamais vu is an event or experience that is familiar but not recognised by the patient. Hallucination is a perception in the absence of external stimulus. Retrograde amnesia is a loss of memory of events that occurred before the onset of amnesia. A delusion is a false personal belief.

4. E

This scenario describes tabes dorsalis, a neurosyphilitic syndrome that results from demyelination of the dorsal roots. It is caused by treponema pallidum and typically presents with dorsal column loss. Mycobacterium tuberculosis causes tuberculosis and Borrelia burgdorferi causes lyme disease. Cryptococcal meningitis causes meningitis and Taenia solium causes neurocysticerocsis.

5. D

A central scotoma suggests a lesion within the macula. Ipsilateral blindness suggests a lesion in the optic nerve and bitemporal hemianopia suggests a lesion in the optic chiasm. Homonymous hemianopia suggests a lesion in the optic tract and left/right superior quadrantanopia suggests a temporal lobe lesion.

6. B

Syringomyelia is where a fluid-filled cyst exists within the spinal cord, which can enlarge and expand into the grey and white matter compressing the tissue of corticospinal and spinothalamic tracts and anterior horn cells. This causes dissociated sensory loss (absent pain and temperature sensation with preserved light touch, vibration and joint-position sense). Option C results from injury to the dorsal column medial lemniscus pathway and option D results from injury to the spinocerebellar tracts.

7. B

This scenario describes the testing of the corneal reflex, which is an involuntary blinking of the eyelids elicited by stimulation of the cornea. The reflex is stimulated by the nasociliary branch of the ophthalmic branch of the trigeminal nerve (sensory response) and the temporal and zygomatic branch of the facial nerve (motor response).

EMQ

This question is based on the various tracts within the central nervous system.

8. C

This scenario describes a lower motor neuron lesion. Lower motor neuron signs indicate that the lesion is either in the anterior horn cell or distal to the anterior horn cell, that is, anterior horn cell, root, plexus or peripheral nerve.

9. I

Decussates in the medulla at the level of the brainstem

10. B

The peripheral nerve travels through the dorsal root ganglion where it synapses (first order neurone) and travels upwards in the dorsal horn neurone and synapses again (second-order neurone) before decussation. Decussation occurs at the level of the spinal cord. It then ascends and synapses at the thalamus (third order neurone).

Head and Neck (Chapter 14)

1.
  a. The facial nerve (cranial nerve VII) is largely motor in function and serves all the muscles of facial expression, therefore if the facial nerve is affected the facial muscles on that side will be weak or completely paralysed (1)
  b. The levator palpebrae superioris (1) is responsible for eye opening. This muscle is innervated by the oculomotor nerve (cranial nerve III), therefore eye opening will be unaffected (1)
  c. Determine if the patient can wrinkle their forehead or not. (1) In lower motor neuron lesion the patient cannot wrinkle their forehead whereas in upper motor neuron lesion the patient can (unless there is bilateral lesion).
  d. The taste to the anterior two-thirds of the tongue is supplied by the chorda tympani, a branch of the facial nerve (1)
  e. The lingual branch of the mandibular division of the trigeminal nerve supplies sensation to anterior two-thirds of the tongue. The glossopharyngeal nerve supplies sensation to the posterior third of the tongue (1)
  f. Second pharyngeal arch (1)
  g. Any one of the following scores one mark: total of three marks.
  Muscles of facial expression
  Stapedius
  Stylohyoid
  Auricular
  Posterior belly of digastric
  Platysma

Cranial nerves may be affected singly or in groups, and knowledge of which nerves are involved helps locate the lesion. Conditions which can affect any cranial nerve:

- Diabetes mellitus
- MS
- Tumours
- Sarcoid
- Vasculitis (e.g. polyarteritis nodosa)
- Systemic lupus erythematosus (SLE)
- Syphilis

2.
  a. Lateral wall – zygomatic bone (1)
     Medial wall – ethmoid bone (1)
  b. Trigeminal nerve (1), maxillary branch (1)
  c. Hyphaema (1)
  d. Proptosis (or exophthalmos) (1)
  e. Aqueous humour is produced by the ciliary body. (1) It first drains through the posterior chamber to enter the anterior chamber. (1) Aqueous humour then exits the eye through the trabecular meshwork into Schlemm's canal (1)
  f. Cerebrospinal fluid (cerebrospinal fluid rhinorrhoea) (1)

This question looks at a potential facial injury and its consequences. It is important to have some knowledge of the bones that make up the cranium and face.

Skull fractures generally result from blunt force or penetrating trauma. Resulting clear fluid draining from the ears or nose is evidence of cerebrospinal fluid leak due to a basal skull fracture. The pterion is a junction between the temporal, frontal, parietal and sphenoid bones. As the thinnest part of the skull, it is a potential point of weakness.

Facial fractures are generally due to trauma as well. Due to their position, the nasal bones are most commonly fractured. The Le Fort system classifies maxillofacial bone fractures based on the bones involved.

3.
  a. Dysphagia is defined as difficulty in swallowing (1)
  b. To the subclavian vein (1)
  c. The thyroid gland is invested in a sheath derived from the pretracheal fascia which holds the gland on to the larynx and trachea. (1) Therefore the thyroid follows the movements of the larynx during swallowing (1)
  d. Superior thyroid artery (1)
     Inferior thyroid artery (1)
  e. A space between the pretracheal and prevertebral fascial layers. (1) The retropharyngeal space extends into the thorax. Therefore, infection in this space can spread to the mediastinal contents (1)

f. The cervical fascia acts to support the viscera of the neck, muscles, blood and lymphatic vessels and deep lymph nodes. (1) It also acts to compartmentalise most structures of the neck and prevents the spread of infections (1)

The fascial layers of the neck have an important clinical significance. Infections that occur deep to the fascia have a well-defined spread.

- Between the investing fascia and visceral part of the pretracheal fascia: infection may spread into the anterior mediastinum.
- Posterior to the prevertebral fascia: erosion through the fascia and into the retropharyngeal space can occur, leading to infections within the mediastinum.

4.
  a. Mastoiditis (1)
  b. Cochlea and vestibular apparatus (1)
  c. Cochlear aqueduct (1)
  d. Infections within the ear can spread via mastoid air cells to cause sub-arachnoid infections (1)
  e. Malleus incus and stapes (1)
  f. Synovial joint. (1) Transmits the sound wave channelled from the external ear-tympanic membrane to the middle ear via the oval window (1)
  g. Any one of the following scores one mark:
     Stapedius
     Tensor tympani
  h. Malleus (1) and incus (1)

This question focuses mainly on the anatomy of the middle ear and its transmission of sound. The ear can be split into the outer, middle and inner parts. Infection can affect any one or all three parts. Middle ear infections can spread to the mastoid air cells and the mastoid process. If this spreads to the middle meningeal fossa, it can cause meningitis.

5.
  a. Glossopharyngeal nerve (1)
     Vagus nerve (1)
  b. Thyroglossal duct (1)
  c. Sternohyoid (1) and sternothyroid (1)
  d. Decreased serum calcium levels (1)
     Increased serum phosphate levels (1)
  e. Chief cells (1)
  f. The left and right recurrent laryngeal nerves. (1) Damage can lead to voice hoarseness and, in severe cases, aphonia and airway obstruction (1)

This question is based on the thyroid and parathyroid glands located in the anterior neck. Thyroxine is produced by the thyroid gland and controlled via negative feedback. The thyroid hormones act on nearly every cell in the body and are essential to proper development and differentiation of all cells in the human body. They are involved in many processes including increasing the basal metabolic rate and affecting protein synthesis.

6.
    a. Palatine tonsils (1)
       Nasopharyngeal tonsils (1)
       Lingual tonsils (1)
    b. Nasopharyngeal tonsils (adenoid) (1)
    c. Middle cranial fossa (1)
    d. Any one of the following scores one mark: total of two marks
       Eustachian tube blockage by accumulation of pus and mucus
       Fluid build-up in the middle ear
       Tympanic membrane perforation
    e. Nasopharynx (via the Eustachian tube) (1) and inner ear via the oval window (1)
    f. The Eustachian tube is relatively narrow and horizontal in children (1)

7.
    a. Synovial joint (1)
    b. Temporomandibular ligament (1)
       Stylomandibular ligament (1)
       Sphenomandibular ligament (1)
    c. The superior compartment allows protraction and retraction of the mandible (1)
       The inferior compartment allows elevation and depression of the mandible (1)
    d. Masseter, temporalis and medial pterygoid. (1) Supplied by mandibular division of the trigeminal nerve (1)
    e. 1st pharyngeal arch (1)
    f. Anterior two-thirds of the tongue (1)

The TMJ is formed by the articulation of the mandible and the temporal bone. The upper part of the joint allows protrusion and retraction of the mandible whereas the lower part of the joint permits opening and closing of the mandible. Dislocation of the TMJ can occur via a blow to the side of the face, or even taking a large bite. The head of the mandible slips out of the mandibular fossa, and is pulled anteriorly.

8.
    a. Ophthalmic artery (1)
    b. Retinal artery occlusion. (1) This is usually as a consequence of embolism (1) secondary to carotid artery disease as a result of atherosclerotic plaques (1)
    c. Optic canal (1)
    d. Any one of the following scores one mark: total of two marks.
       Central retinal vein occlusion
       Optic neuritis
       Ischaemic optic neuropathy
       Eye and optic nerve tumours

    e. Cataracts (1)

      Macular degeneration (1)

    f. Loss of innervation to levator palpebrae superioris muscle which elevates and retracts the upper eyelid (1)

This question focuses on the eye. Sudden loss of vision is an ophthalmological emergency and requires immediate referral to the eye emergency department. Optic nerve fibres divide and cross over at the optic chiasm. Clinical patterns can help you locate the site of the visual defect:

- Loss of vision in one eye – the problem is the eye itself or in the optic nerve before the optic chiasm.
- Bitemporal hemianopia – caused by lesions compressing the optic chiasm such as a pituitary tumour.
- Homonymous hemianopia – the lesion is somewhere between the optic chiasm and the occiput.

9.

    a. Tumour eroding the superior part of the sympathetic chain, causing loss of sympathetic innervation to the levator palpebrae superioris (1), to the face (anhidrosis), vasodilatation (red), miosis (constricted pupil) and the smooth muscle part of levator palpebrae superioris (ptosis)

    b. Interruption of sympathetic innervation to dilator pupillae as a consequence of tumour. (1) Right pupil will be larger (1)

    c. The light reflex would be normal, (1) although with less constriction on the left as the pupil is already more constricted (1)

    d. Hemipalsy on the left (1) due to injury to the recurrent laryngeal nerve which supplies all the intrinsic muscles of the larynx except the cricothyroid (1)

    e. Due to palsy of the larynx (1) and paralysis of diaphragm (1) as the tumour compresses on the recurrent laryngeal nerve and the phrenic nerve respectively

    f. Squamous cell (1)

This question focuses on Horner's syndrome, which results from disruption of the sympathetic nerves that supply the eye. Its associated with a triad:

- Partial ptosis
- Miosis
- Anhidrosis

Management involves diagnosis and treatment of the underlying condition. One potential cause for Horner's syndrome might be an apical lung tumour. This is a second-order nerve lesion.

10.

    a. Roof and posterior wall of nasopharynx (1)

    b. Pseudostratified columnar epithelium (1)

c. Eustachian tube (1)
d. Any one of the following scores one mark: total of three marks.
　Obstructive sleep apnoea
　Obstructive adenoid hyperplasia
　Middle ear infection
　Cardiopulmonary complications, for example, pulmonary hypertension
e. Any one of the following scores one mark:
　Adenovirus
　Rhinovirus
　Paramyxovirus
f. Any one of the following scores one mark:
　Haemophilus influenzae – gram negative
　Group A beta-haemolytic streptococcus – gram positive
　Staphylococcus aureus – gram positive
　Moraxella catarrhalis – gram negative
　Streptococcus pneumoniae – gram positive
g. Any one of the following scores one mark: total of two marks.
　Bleeding
　Velopharyngeal insufficiency
　Torticollis
　Nasopharyngeal stenosis

This question's focus was around the lymphatic tissue of the neck. **Waldeyer's tonsillar ring** refers to the collection of lymphatic tissue surrounding the upper pharynx. The palatine tonsils are part of this ring and can become **inflamed** due to a viral or bacterial infection. If an infection spreads to the **peritonsillar tissue,** it can cause an abscess to form. This is known as **quinsy**. It is treated with draining of the abscess and antibiotics. Quinsy can potentially cause obstruction of the pharynx.

Another clinically important lymph node to be aware of is Virchow's node. This is located in the left supraclavicular fossa and when enlarged, may indicate the presence of a gastric cancer that has spread through the lymph vessels. This is because this node receives lymphatic drainage from the abdominal cavity.

MCQ

1. B

The cavernous sinus is located on either side of the pituitary fossa and body of the sphenoid bone and becomes a potential route of infection due to its connections with the facial and cerebral veins. The spread of infection into the cavernous sinus can result in central nervous system infection or cavernous sinus thrombosis.

2. E

The thyroid gland is invested in a sheath derived from the pretracheal fascia. This holds the gland on to the larynx and trachea therefore the thyroid follows the movements of the larynx during swallowing.

3. A

The muscles of mastication (masseter, temporalis, medial and lateral pterygoid) are innervated by the mandibular branch of the trigeminal nerve. Other facial muscles are innervated by the facial nerve.

4. C

The innervation of taste and sensation is different for the anterior and posterior parts of the tongue. Sensation to the anterior two-thirds of the tongue is via the lingual branch of the mandibular division of the trigeminal nerve whereas the taste is via the chorda tympani branch of the facial nerve. Sensation and taste to the posterior third of the tongue is via the glossopharyngeal nerve.

5. D

Superior orbital fissure syndrome is a neurological disorder expressed by altered functions of nerves passing through the superior orbital fissure due to fracture within the region of the fissure. Ophthalmoplegia occurs due to paresis of cranial nerves III, IV and VI. Ptosis and exophthalmos occurs due to disruption of the venous drainage and mydriasis results from loss of parasympathetic innervation.

6. B

The pterygopalatine ganglion is located in the pterygopalatine fossa and supplies the lacrimal gland, paranasal sinuses, glands of the mucosa of the nasal cavity and pharynx, the gingiva and the mucous membrane and glands of the hard palate. The ciliary ganglion is associated with the oculomotor nerve and the submandibular ganglion is associated with the lingual nerve and chorda tympani. The otic ganglion is associated with the glossopharyngeal nerve.

7. A

The cricothyroid muscle is one of the muscles of the pharynx and aids phonation. It is the only laryngeal muscle supplied by the superior laryngeal branch of the vagus nerve. Options B–E are innervated by the recurrent laryngeal nerve.

EMQ

This question is based on the various structures within the skull

8. I

Jugular foramen syndrome (or Vernet's syndrome) is characterised by the paresis of cranial nerves IX, X and XI resulting in various symptoms and signs such dysphagia, dysarthria, hoarseness of voice, loss of taste on posterior third of tongue and paresis of soft palate, uvula, pharynx and larynx. In addition to these cranial nerves the foramen also contains the internal jugular vein.

9. G

An epidural haematoma typically results from a blow to the side of the head. The pterion region overlies the middle meningeal artery which is prone to injury. This artery runs through the foramen spinosum.

10. D

Bell's palsy results from dysfunction of the facial nerve. The course of the facial nerve is complex and involves both intracranial and extracranial routes. The intracranial course starts in the pons and travels through the internal acoustic meatus and enters the facial canal. Within the canal the nerve forms the geniculate ganglion and gives rise to the greater petrosal nerve, nerve to the stapedius and the chorda tympani. Finally the nerve exits the canal via the stylomastoid foramen. The extracranial course involves the entrance into the parotid gland where it terminates by splitting into five branches (temporal, zygomatic, buccal, marginal mandibular and cervical).

Clinical Pharmacology (Chapter 15)

1.
    a. Ciclosporin binds to the cytoplasmic protein cyclophilin T lymphocytes. (1) This complex of ciclosporin and cyclophilin inhibits calcineurin, which is normally responsible for activating the transcription of inter-leukin-2. This leads to a reduced function of T cells (1)
    b. Any one of the following scores one mark: total of two marks.
       Gut motility
       First pass metabolism
       Drug destruction by gut or bacterial enzymes
       Splanchnic blood flow
       Lipophilicity
       Pharmaceutical preparation
       pH
    c. Therapeutic – cyclooxygenase-2 (COX-2) (1)
       Adverse drug reactions – cyclooxygenase-1 (COX-1) (1)
    d. Pharmacological actions for the majority of NSAIDs are via competitive inhibition of cyclooxygenase-1 and cycooxygenase-2. (1) Occupation of these enzyme channels competes with arachidonic acid site occupation thereby reduces formation of prostaglandins and thromboxane (1)
    e. Any one of the following scores one mark: total of two marks.
       EP1 (Gq) – sensitise peripheral nociception
       EP2 (Gs) – sensitise central nociception
       EP3 (Gi) – increase heat production and reduce heat loss

This question focuses on immunosuppression and disease modifying therapy in rheumatoid arthritis. Examples of disease modifying anti-rheumatic drugs include methotrexate, sulfasalazine, anti-TNF agents and rituximab. Immunosuppressants include corticosteroids, azathioprine, ciclosporin, tacrolimus and mycophenolate mofetil. Ciclosporin and tacrolimus are known as calcineurin inhibitors and are active against helper T cells preventing the production of IL-2 via calcineurin inhibition. Some adverse effects include nephrotoxicity, hypertension, hyperlipidaemia, gingival hyperplasia and hyperuricemia. Methotrexate is the gold-standard treatment for rheumatoid arthritis. This drug works by competitively and reversibly inhibiting dihydrofolate reductase therefore inhibiting DNA, RNA and protein synthesis.

2.
 a. Metabolised to morphine (1) in the liver by cytochrome P450 2D6 (1)
 b. Delta (1)
  Kappa (1)
  Mu (1)
 c. They increase potassium outflow therefore decrease excitability (1)
 d. ED_{50}: the dose that produces a therapeutic effect in 50% of the population that takes it (1)
  LD_{50}: the dose of a substance required to kill 50% of the test population (1)
 e. Respiratory depression (1)
 f. Naloxone (1)

This question focuses on opioids. These can be classified into endogenous and exogenous. Endogenous opioids are distributed in specific parts of the central nervous system and peripheral nervous system. There are three major groups consisting of endorphins, enkephalins and dynorphins. Exogenous opioids are natural, semi-synthetic or synthetic agents that act on endogenous opioid receptors (mainly mu, kappa and delta). These receptors are all g protein-coupled receptors. Binding at mu receptors results in an increased outward flux of potassium resulting in decreased excitability. Binding at kappa receptors causes a decreased influx of calcium and binding at mu, and delta receptors result in decreased cAMP synthesis. Binding at different receptor subtypes results in different actions, for example, μ_1 is responsible for the main analgesic effect whereas μ_2 causes adverse drug reactions such as nausea and vomiting, constipation, drowsiness, miosis, respiratory depression and hypotension.

3.
 a. Paracetamol is metabolised in the liver by conjugation with glucuronic acid and sulfuric acid. (1) Hepatotoxic metabolites (NAPQI) produced by cytochrome P450 is detoxified by conjugation with glutathione (1)
 b. In overdose, the conjugation of NAPQI is saturated leading to increasing toxic levels of NAPQI (1)
 c. Treatment is determined by plotting the measured plasma paracetamol concentration against the time since ingestion commenced, using a nomogram. (1) Patients with a plasma paracetamol concentration above the nomogram line require treatment. (1) However, patients with clinical features of hepatic injury or serious toxicity (150 mg/kg in any 24-hour period) can be commenced on treatment before paracetamol levels are available (1)

   d. Intravenous N-acetylcysteine (2)
   e. One mark for labelling of axis
      One mark for shape of curve

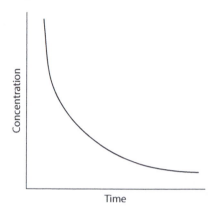

This question focuses on drug metabolism. This involves phase I enzymes that catalyse the modification of existing functional groups in drug molecules (oxidation reactions). Phase II involves conjugating enzymes which facilitate the addition of endogenous molecules such as sulfate, glucuronic acid and glutathione. The end products of conjugation are water-soluble therefore enabling rapid elimination from the body. Paracetamol is metabolised to sulfate (30%) and glucuronide (60%). It also undergoes cytochrome P450 oxidation into NAPQI which is conjugated with glutathione to inactive metabolites cysteine/mercapturic acid (10%). In substantial overdose, the conjugation of NAPQI is saturated leading to increasing toxic levels of NAPQI. Therefore treatment is to replace glutathione.

4.
   a. Olanzapine (antipsychotic) has an antagonistic effect to both dopamine D_2 receptors (1) and 5-HT_{2A} serotonin receptors. (1) Olanzapine has a higher affinity for 5-HT_{2A} serotonin receptors than D_2 dopamine receptors.
   b. Parkinson's disease (1)
   c. Any one of the following scores one mark: total of two marks.
      Weight gain
      Postural hypotension
      Drowsiness
      Diabetes
   d. Any one of the following scores one mark: total of two marks.
      Withdrawn or restless
      Noisy
      Tardive dyskinesia
      Poor eye contact
      Apathy

   e. Selective serotonin reuptake inhibitor. (1) Inhibits reuptake of serotonin therefore serotonin stays longer in the synaptic gap and hence stimulates receptors (1)

   f. Use of selective serotonin reuptake inhibitors has been linked with suicidal ideation hence patients should be monitored for suicidal behaviour, self-harm or hostility (1)

5.

   a. Any one of the following scores one mark: total of two marks.
Alcohol
Menstruation
Missed medication
Stress
Lack of sleep

   b. All types of partial seizures and generalised tonic–clonic seizures (1)

   c. Anticonvulsant (1)

   d. Carbamazepine is a voltage gated sodium channel blocker. (1) It binds to these when the channel is depolarised. This prolongs the inactivation state and prevents further depolarisation (1)

   e. It is a strong cytochrome P450 enzyme inducer. (1) Therefore it can increase the clearance of other drugs and also reduce its own half-life if given repeatedly (1)

   f. Sodium valproate (1) because it is associated with the highest risk of major and minor congenital malformations and long-term neurodevelopmental effects (1)

This question focuses on psychopharmacology. Central nervous system drugs can act as simulators (agonists) or blockers (antagonists) of neurotransmitter receptors. Antidepressants include selective serotonin reuptake inhibitors (first-line treatment for moderate to severe depression), tricyclics (block reuptake of serotonin and noradrenaline), and non-selective monoamine reuptake inhibitors. Drugs used to treat schizophrenia include typical and atypical antipsychotics and clozapine. Advantages of atypical antipsychotics are fewer side effects, different available preparations and differing side-effect profiles that can be matched to patient characteristics. This group of drugs is now used as first-line treatment in schizophrenia. Typical antipsychotics are well known for their side effects and toxicity, for example, extrapyramidal side effects (parkinsonism, acute dystonia, akathasia, tardive dyskinesia) and neuroleptic malignant syndrome (severe rigidity, hyperthermia, autonomic lability and increased creatine phosphokinase). Benzodiazepines can be used to treat anxiety and work by acting as full agonists at GABA-benzodiazepine receptors leading to enhancement of GABA.

6.

   a. Any one of the following scores one mark: total of two marks.
Ulcerative colitis: continuous inflammation, mucosa shows erythema, friability and frank superficial bleeding, pseudopolyps.

Crohn's disease: aphthous ulcer, cobblestone appearance of mucosa, transmural inflammation, strictures and fistulas

b. Ulcerative colitis (1)
c. Erythema nodosum (1)
d. Any one of the following scores one mark:
   Pyoderma gangrenosum
   Aphthous stomatitis
   Vasculitis
   Psoriasis
e. Immunosuppressants like steroids and azathioprine reduce the body's ability to fight off common infections (1)
f. There is an inflammatory response in the body where macrophages are stimulated to release interleukin-1 (IL-1). IL-1 increases the production of prostaglandin E2 (PGE2) by cyclooxygenase in the hypothalamus. (1) PGE2 acts on prostaglandin EP3 receptors which causes increased heat production regulated by the thermoregulatory centre (1)
g. Any one of the following drug scores one mark and another one mark for correct mechanism: total of two marks
   Non-steroidal anti-inflammatory drugs – blocks the COX-2 pathway in the synthesis of PGE2.
   Paracetamol – considered to be a weak inhibitor of prostaglandin synthesis.

This question focuses on non-steroidal anti-inflammatory drugs (NSAIDs). Its main therapeutic effects are analgesia, anti-inflammatory and antipyretic. The pharmacological action for nearly all NSAIDs are via competitive inhibition of COX-1 and COX-2. Occupation of COX-1/2 hydrophobic channel by NSAID competes with arachidonic acid site occupation. Its main therapeutic effects are achieved via COX-2 inhibition. Inhibition of COX-1 constitutive prostaglandin synthesis is responsible for side effects. Its main side effects are related to the gastrointestinal (GI) tract including stomach pain, nausea, heartburn, gastric bleeding and ulceration. This occurs because NSAIDs reduce gastric COX-1 prostaglandin E2 production therefore reducing cytoprotective mucus secretion throughout the GI tract, increasing acid secretion and reducing mucosal blood flow.

7.
   a. Protein pump inhibitors bind irreversibly to hydrogen-potassium ATPase (proton pumps) on gastric parietal cells (1) and block the secretion of hydrogen ions (1)
   b. Any one of the following drug scores one mark and another mark for correct mechanism.
      H_2 receptor antagonists (e.g. ranitidine) – block the action of histamine on histamine H_2 receptors of the parietal cells, thereby decreasing stomach acid production.
      Antacids – contain alkaline ions that neutralise stomach gastric acid.
   c. Any one of the following scores one mark: total of two marks.
      Nausea and vomiting

Abdominal pain
Flatulence
Diarrhoea
Constipation

d. Any one of the following scores one mark: total of four marks.
Side effects
Medical device adverse incidents
Defective medicines
Counterfeit or fake medicines, or medical devices
Safety concerns for e-cigarettes or their refill containers

This question focuses on drugs affecting acid secretion. Proton pump inhibitors are acid-activated prodrugs that target ATPase. They inhibit gastric acid secretion by blocking the hydrogen-potassium adenosine triphosphatase enzyme system (proton pump) of gastric parietal cells. The action is delayed as not all pumps are active all of the time therefore maximum efficacy occurs after two to 3 days. Main side effects associated with this class of drugs include gastrointestinal disturbance (nausea, vomiting, abdominal pain, flatulence, diarrhoea, constipation) and headache. Histamine-2 receptor antagonists reduce gastric output as a result of histamine H_2-receptor blockade. Alginate taken in combination with an antacid increases the viscosity of stomach contents and can protect the oesophageal mucosa from acid reflux. Some alginate-containing preparations form a viscous gel ('raft') that floats on the surface of the stomach contents, thereby reducing reflux symptoms.

8.

a. Any one of the following scores one mark: total of four marks.

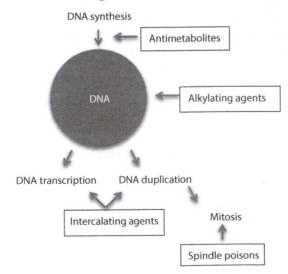

b. Any one of the following scores one mark: total of two marks.
Age
General state of health (performance status)

Co-morbidities (heart, liver, kidney disease)
Psychosocial status
Previous cancer treatments (response and adverse effects)
c. It inhibits formation and increase in polymerisation of spindle in meta-phase (1) during mitosis therefore cells are unable to proliferate (1)
d. One mark for correct shape of curve.

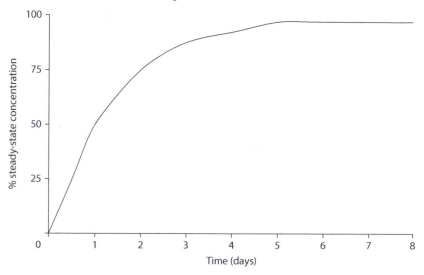

e. Day 2 (1)

This question focuses on cancer chemotherapy. Alkylating agents work by formation of platinated inter- and intrastrand adducts resulting in inhibition of DNA synthesis. Antimetabolites induce cell death during the S phase of cell growth when incorporated into RNA and DNA or inhibit enzymes required for nucleic acid production. Spindle poisons such as vinca alkaloids work by causing inhibition of polymerisation of tubulin into microtubules. Chemotherapy is associated with a wide range of side effects such as vomiting, alopecia and mucositis. Toxicity involves the skin which can present as thrombophlebitis of veins and extravasation. Cardiotoxicity, for example, cardiomyopathy is associated with doxorubicin and arrhythmias can be caused by cyclophosphamide and etoposide. Pulmonary fibrosis is associated with many drugs such as bleomycin, mitomycin C and cyclophosphamide. Haematological toxicity is the most frequent dose limiting and the most frequent cause of death from toxicity.

MCQ

1. B

This scenario describes acute cholecystitis, an acute inflammation of the gallbladder usually associated with impacted gallstones or biliary sludge at the neck of the gallbladder or cystic duct. Opioids are usually required for pain relief. The classic teaching is that morphine is not the agent of choice because of the possibility of increasing tone at the sphincter of Oddi. Pethidine is therefore the preferred choice due to its opioid effect as well its anticholinergic properties therefore it is least likely to cause spasm of the sphincter.

2. D

Cyclophosphamide is an alkylating agent that works by forming inter- and intrastrand adducts leading to inhibition of DNA synthesis. Cyclophosphamide is metabolised to its metabolite acrolein which is toxic to bladder epithelium leading to haemorrhagic cystitis.

3. A

This patient presents with a low potassium level. Therefore, it is appropriate to use a potassium sparing diuretic, that is, spironolactone. Loop diuretics (furosemide and bumetanide) and thiazides (bendroflumethiazide and indapamide) cause hypokalaemia.

4. E

This scenario describes a simple urinary tract infection. The majority of these infections are caused by Escherichia coli (E-coli). It is recommended by NICE to offer an antibiotic to all women with a suspected urinary tract infection a 3-day course of either nitrofurantoin or trimethoprim. Azithromycin can be used to treat chlamydia and gonorrhoea infections. Doxycycline can be used to treat chlamydia infection. Fluconazole is an antifungal and used to treat vaginal candidiasis. Cefotaxime can be used to treat urinary tract infections but typically not first line and can be used to treat gonorrhoea.

5. B

Diazepam is a benzodiazepine and the antidote to treat this is flumazenil. Naloxone is used to treat opioid overdose. Protamine is used to treat heparin overdose. Deferoxamine is used to treat iron poisoning and glucagon is used to treat beta-blocker poisoning.

6. C

Cimetidine is an H_2 receptor antagonist and an example of an hepatic enzyme inhibitor. Therefore, administration of warfarin with cimetidine will result in enhanced activity of warfarin hence an increased INR reading.

7. B

The time to reach steady state is defined by the elimination half-life of the drug. After one half-life, you will have reached 50% of steady state. After two half-lives, you will have reached 75% of steady state, and after three half-lives you will have reached 87.5% of steady state. It usually takes five half-lives to reach steady state. Therefore if a half-live is 8 hours it would be expected that a 75% steady state would be reached in 16 hours.

EMQ

This question is based on the a range of medications to treat different conditions.

8. B

Macrolides (e.g. erythromycin) interfere with protein synthesis by reversibly binding to the 50S subunit of the ribosome. They appear to bind at the donor site, thus preventing the translocation necessary to keep the peptide chain growing.

9. E

Rifampicin is a potent enzyme inducer therefore reduces the effect of the oral contraceptive pill. Faculties of sexual and reproductive healthcare now recommend that no additional precautions are required to maintain contraceptive efficacy when using antibiotics that are not enzyme inducers with combined hormonal methods for durations of 3 weeks or less.

10. G

Gentamicin, an aminoglycoside works by irreversibly binding the 30S subunit of the bacterial ribosome, interrupting protein synthesis. Significant side effects include nephrotoxicity and ototoxicity.

Society and Medicine (Chapter 16)

1.
   a. Incidence: Number of new cases of a disease in a defined population during a defined time period (1)
      Prevalence: Proportion of people affected with a disease in a defined population at a particular point in time (1)
   b. Eight new cases of MS (1) per 10 000 people per year (1)
      Incidence rate – new events / (person × time) (years)
      Therefore incidence rate – 600 / (500 000 × 1.5) – 0.00008, that is, 8 cases of MS per 10,000 people per year.
   c. It would reduce the prevalence but not the incidence (1)
   d. Likely due to people who suffer from MS are alive for longer (1)
      Prevalence can increase as a consequence of increased incidence (1)
   e. An odds ratio of 1.5 means that with the new treatment for MS you are 50% more likely to be alive 10 years after diagnosis compared to conventional treatment. (1) There is insufficient evidence to suggest any statistically significant difference between the new and old treatment as the confidence interval includes 1.0 (1)
   f. All patients that were enrolled and randomly allocated to treatment are included within the analysis and are analysed in the groups to which they were originally randomised. This is regardless of whether they complete the trial or not (1)

This question focuses on measuring disease in populations. Incidence rate measures new cases whereas prevalence measures existing cases. The relationship between incidence and prevalence can be affected by various factors. An increased prevalence can be the result of an increased incidence and the fact that patients are living longer. A decreased prevalence can be due to curing more patients or the fact that more patients are dying. Incidence rate ratio allows the comparison of incidence rates between groups with different levels of exposure but can also be used to compare the effects of two treatments and decide which is the best.

2.
- a. No. (1) Smoking has increased within the general population and therefore is likely to have increased in the population of people recently diagnosed with a bladder cancer. In this case, smoking is a compounding factor (1)
- b. Case-control study (1)
  Any one of the following scores one mark: total of two marks.
  Quicker and cheaper
  Able to study several exposure factors simultaneously
  Efficient for rare diseases or diseases with a long latency period between exposure and disease manifestation
- c. 2.5 (1)
  Incidence rate ratio – incidence rate 1 / incidence rate 2
  Incidence 1 – 3 in 100,000 = 0.00003
  Incidence 2 – 12 in 1,000,000 = 0.000012
  Therefore incidence ratio = 0.00003 / 0.000012 = 2.5
- d. 0.7 (1) to 8.75 (1)
  Lower 95% confidence interval – observed value / error factor
  Upper 95% confidence interval – observed value × error factor
- e. Yes. (1) Because the stated hypothesis of incidence rate ratio of 1.0 lies within the 95% confidence interval therefore $p > 0.05$ and we cannot reject the hypothesis (1)

This question focuses on case-control studies. This is an analytical study that starts by identifying a group of cases and a suitable group of non-cases (controls) followed by investigating exposures of interests in the past. Groups are then compared using an odds ratio, that is, comparing the odds of having been exposed in the cases with the odds of having been exposed in the controls. Key issues that lie within a case-control study is selection bias, information bias and confounding factors. Case-control studies have an advantage over cohort studies by being quicker therefore relatively cheaper, and also able to study a range of exposures for a single outcome or disease.

3.
- a. The 95% confidence interval does not include 1 and the p value is below 0.05, therefore we can reject the null hypothesis with over 95%

certainty and the result is statistically significant. (1) An odds ratio of 2.23 indicates that the cases in this study are two times more likely to be exposed than the controls (1), that is, patients taking conjugated oestrogens are 2.23 times more likely to develop endometrial cancer compared to patients not taking conjugated oestrogens. However, this only shows an association, and temporal sequence (exposure precedes disease) cannot be established (1)

b. Any one of the following scores one mark: total of two marks.
   Advantages:
   Quicker and cheaper
   Can study range of exposures
   Good for rare outcomes, for example, rare diseases
   Any one of the following scores one mark: total of two marks.
   Disadvantages:
   Not good for rare exposures
   Prone to information and selection bias
   Can be difficult to eliminate reverse causality

c. Denial, anger, bargaining, depression (2)

d. Set clear quality requirements for care and offer strategies, and support to help organisations achieve these (1)

This question focuses on case-control studies again. Refer to summary in question 2.

4.

a. Obtain the consent of the parent or responsible adult when collecting personal data (1)
   Take special care with the questions asked taking into account their age and level of maturity (1)

b. No, (1) because when compared to the rest of the country this is not age adjusted, that is, age is a confounding factor (1)

c. By conducting a cohort study (1) that allows to compare risks based on exposures (1)

d. Yes. (1) A randomised controlled trial aims to give a fair comparison of effect and safety of a clinical intervention. It helps avoid problems of confounding using stratification but has problems associated with loss to follow-up. (1) A systematic review is an overview of primary studies that uses explicit and reproducible methods that limits bias by identifying and rejecting studies. (1) Conclusions are more reliable and accurate because of the methods used (1)

This question focuses on the review of evidence. Healthcare services and interventions should be based on best available evidence. A systematic review is an extremely credible source of evidence. It is defined as an overview of primary studies that used explicit and reproducible methods. Key aspects are that is explicit, transparent and reproducible therefore unbiased and objective. A meta-analysis is a quantitative synthesis of the results of two or more primary studies that addressed the same hypothesis in the same way. It aims to facilitate the synthesis of a large number of study results, systematically collate study results, reduce problems of interpretation due to variations in sampling, and quantify effect sizes and their uncertainty as a pooled estimate. However, problems associated with meta-analysis include heterogeneity between studies, variable quality of the studies and publication bias in the selection of studies.

5.
  a. Any one of the following scores one mark:
     Familial adenomatous polyposis
     Lynch syndrome
     Turcot syndrome
     Peutz-Jeghers syndrome
  b. Prospective – exposure precedes outcome. Patient is disease-free at the start, followed up over time and the outcome is observed (1)
     Retrospective – exposure precedes outcome but data is taken from historical records, that is, past exposure, and it is observed whether disease was present or not (1)
  c. A vegetarian diet has a 95% confidence interval of adjusted risk of 0.65 to 0.86 which does not include null hypothesis. This suggests $p<0.05$ and the difference is not due to chance. (1) It is statistically significant to reject the null hypothesis and we are 95% sure the relative risk is between 0.65 and 0.86 (1)
  d. There is a reduction in risk. (1) However, the 95% confidence interval includes the null hypothesis which means $p>0.05$ and the reduction could be due to chance. So it is not statistically significant, therefore the null hypothesis cannot be rejected (1)
  e. The clinical condition of a participant may necessitate their removal from the trial (1)
     Participants may choose to withdraw from the trial (1)
  f. It is a factor that relates both to exposure and outcome, but does not lie in the casual pathway itself (1)

This question focuses on randomised control trials (RCTs). This is a clinical trial in which interventions are studies, in contrast to observational studies. Steps involved in conducting an RCT involve identifying, recruiting, consenting and maintaining two comparable groups of participants. One group is then allocated to treatment whereas the other group is given standard treatment. These groups are then followed up with the aim to maintain all participants in the trial. Groups are then assessed using the same criteria and outcomes are compared in both groups. RCT helps to minimise confounding factors using stratification. Clinical trials should be analysed on an intention-to-treat basis, which is when all people in a trial group are included in the analysis regardless of whether they took a treatment or not. This preserves true randomisation and eliminates confounding factors.

MCQ

1. D

Sensitivity is the ability of a test to detect the presence of a disease in those who truly have the disease. It is calculated as the number of people with a disease who test positive (true positive) divided by the total number of people who have the disease (true positive + false negative). In this case, sensitivity equals 150 / (150 + 70) = 68%.

Option A – positive predictive value which equals true positive divided by true positive + false positive
Option B – negative predictive value which equals false negative divided by false negative + true negative
Option C – specificity which equals true negative divided by false positive + true negative
Option E – prevalence which equals true positive + false negative divided by total number of people tested

2. B

Specificity refers to how well a test identifies persons who do not have the disease. It is calculated by true negatives divided by true negatives + false positives. In this example, 1050 people do not have Crohn's disease and 700 of these people have a negative test.

Option A – sensitivity
Option C – negative predictive value
Option D – positive predictive value

3. A

95% of a normally distributed population will fall between plus or minus 1.96 standard deviations (approximately 2) from the mean. Therefore approximately 2.5% of the population will have an HDL level 2 standard deviations or more above the mean, and 2.5% of the population will have an HDL level 2 standard deviations or more below the mean. Therefore, 2.5% of 100 are 2.5 people.

4. E

Prevalence is the proportion of a population that are new and old cases at a given time. It can be measured at a particular point in time (point prevalence) or over a specified period of time (period prevalence). In this scenario, prevalence equals 60 divided by 200,000 = 0.0003. To give the rate per 100,000 we need to multiply 0.0003 by 100,000 = 30 per 100,000.

5. C

This is an example of case-control study which therefore uses odds ratio for comparison. Odds ratio is a common measure of the size of an effect and may be reported in case-control studies, cohort studies or clinical trials. The odds ratio is the ratio between the odds of the treated group and the odds of the control group.

6. E

Analysis of Variance is a hypothesis-testing technique used to test the equality of two or more population (or treatment) means by examining the variances of samples that are taken. ANOVA allows one to determine whether the differences between the samples are simply due to random error or whether there are systematic treatment effects that cause the mean in one group to differ from the mean in another.

7. B

Incidence is the rate of new cases of the disease. It is generally reported as the number of new cases occurring within a period of time. Prevalence is the actual number of cases alive, with the disease either during a period of time (period prevalence) or at a particular date in time (point prevalence).

EMQ

This question is based on the various types of study and statistical analysis.

8. E

A confounder is a factor that is associated with both the exposure and the disease of interest, for example, age and sex. This can be eliminated via randomised controlled trials, which avoids problems of confounding using stratification.

9. B

A cohort study starts with disease-free individuals who then are followed up to see who develops the disease. It can be designed as retrospective or prospective.

10. H

A funnel plot is a graph designed to identify the existence of publication bias and is commonly used in systematic reviews and meta-analysis. If publication bias is present the plot is asymmetrical, and if there is no publication bias the plot is symmetrical.

Index